Selenium-Rich Products: Their Development and Regulation of Human Health

Selenium-Rich Products: Their Development and Regulation of Human Health

Guest Editor

Jiaqiang Huang

MDPI

Basel • Beijing • Wuhan • Barcelona • Belgrade • Novi Sad • Cluj • Manchester

Guest Editor
Jiaqiang Huang
Department of Nutrition and Health
China Agricultural University
Beijing
China

Editorial Office
MDPI AG
Grosspeteranlage 5
4052 Basel, Switzerland

This is a reprint of the Special Issue, published open access by the journal *Nutrients* (ISSN 2072-6643), freely accessible at: https://www.mdpi.com/journal/nutrients/special_issues/99Y45MJ4MC

For citation purposes, cite each article independently as indicated on the article page online and as indicated below:

Lastname, A.A.; Lastname, B.B. Article Title. *Journal Name* **Year**, *Volume Number*, Page Range.

ISBN 978-3-7258-7661-7 (Hbk)
ISBN 978-3-7258-7662-4 (PDF)
https://doi.org/10.3390/books978-3-7258-7662-4

Contents

About the Editor

Jiaqiang Huang

Jiaqiang Huang is an Professor and Ph.D. supervisor in the Department of Nutrition and Health at China Agricultural University, Beijing, China. His research focuses on the biological roles of selenium and selenoproteins, oxidative stress regulation in livestock, and the development of selenium-enriched products. He has led over 15 research projects, including grants from the National Natural Science Foundation of China and the National Key R&D Program. Dr. Huang has published more than 20 SCI-indexed papers as first author or corresponding author in renowned journals such as *Advanced Science*, *Journal of Nutrition*, *Redox Biology*, and *Nutrients*. He also serves as a youth editorial board member, guest editor, and invited reviewer for several international journals.

Preface

The idea for this Special Issue originated from the growing recognition that selenium, while indispensable for human health, operates within a narrow window of efficacy. The global prevalence of selenium deficiency, coupled with the potential toxicity of excess intake, calls for a deeper understanding of how selenium-rich products can be developed and applied safely. This Reprint brings together a collection of studies that not only advance our knowledge of selenium biology but also translate these insights into practical applications in food innovation and disease prevention.

The contributions in this volume encompass a broad research spectrum, ranging from mechanistic studies that elucidate selenium's roles in antioxidant defense, radiation protection, and metabolic regulation, to translational investigations into selenium-enriched products derived from plant sources and nano-formulations. A particular strength of this collection lies in its emphasis on the precision assessment of selenium nutritional status, with erythrocyte selenium emerging as a promising long-term biomarker for guiding personalized supplementation. These findings collectively underscore the importance of balancing efficacy and safety in selenium intervention.

We are grateful to all the authors who contributed their outstanding research to this issue, and to the reviewers who dedicated their time and expertise to ensure the quality of the manuscripts. Special thanks go to the editorial team at MDPI for their continuous support throughout the process. We hope that this compilation will inspire further investigations into the precise roles of selenium in nutrition and health, ultimately contributing to evidence-based dietary strategies worldwide.

Jiaqiang Huang
Guest Editor

nutrients

MDPI

Editorial

Towards Precision and Balance in Selenium Nutrition: From Innovation to Application

Jiaqiang Huang * and Kongdi Zhu

Beijing Advanced Innovation Center for Food Nutrition and Human Health, Department of Nutrition and Health, China Agricultural University, Beijing 100083, China
* Correspondence: jqhuang@cau.edu.cn

Selenium (Se) is an essential trace element for human health, primarily functioning through its incorporation into selenoproteins, which play critical roles in antioxidant defense, immune regulation, and thyroid hormone metabolism [1,2]. While Se deficiency remains a global public health concern linked to various pathologies [3], the safe and effective dietary supplementation of Se continues to be a central focus in nutritional and food science. This Special Issue, "Se-Rich Products: Their Development and Regulation of Human Health," compiles cutting-edge research that not only showcases innovative pathways for developing Se-enriched products but also delves into the complex mechanisms by which Se maintains health and counteracts disease. Collectively, these studies converge on a core theme: the dual imperatives of balance and precision are paramount to realizing the full health benefits of Se intervention.

The contributions in this issue deepen our understanding of the Se-health nexus from multiple dimensions. First, regarding biological mechanisms, several studies elucidate the role of Se in protection against specific environmental and metabolic stressors. Zhang et al. [4] systematically delineate the mechanisms through which Se and selenoproteins exert radioprotective effects via antioxidant actions, DNA repair, and immune enhancement, providing a theoretical foundation for developing radioprotective agents. Concurrently, the study by Li et al. [5] innovatively reveals the mediating role of oxidative stress (marked by albumin and vitamin D) in the association between dietary Se intake and cognitive function in middle-aged and older adults. This work directly links Se's antioxidant properties to neurological outcomes, offering fresh insights for nutritional strategies aimed at mitigating cognitive decline. The theme of precision is further exemplified by studies on specific selenoproteins. An emerging study [6] reveals a novel mechanism by which the selenoprotein I regulates ferroptosis in colitis and colorectal cancer, independent of the well-known suppressor GPX4. Expanding this understanding of selenoprotein specificity, research on Selenoprotein V (SELENOV) has uncovered its critical in vivo functions. Studies demonstrate that SELENOV knockout in mice leads to increased fat accumulation, attenuated energy expenditure, and heightened susceptibility to pro-oxidant-induced liver injury and endoplasmic reticulum stress [7,8]. These findings establish SELENOV as a novel regulator of lipid metabolism, thermogenesis, and cellular redox resilience, highlighting the diverse and targeted roles individual selenoproteins play in metabolic health and stress response.

Complementing these mechanistic advances, the field is witnessing significant innovation in the development and validation of novel Se-rich products and sophisticated delivery systems. For instance, Zhu et al. [9] demonstrated the development of a functional product using the Se hyperaccumulator Cardamine violifolia, while concurrently highlighting the

 https://doi.org/10.3390/nu18020320

critical issue of co-accumulated heavy metals. This case underscores the imperative for rigorous safety assessments throughout the development of natural Se sources, a point reinforced by broader reviews advocating for full "soil-to-table" chain control to ensure safety and efficacy [10]. Beyond plants, the biotransformation capabilities of food-grade microorganisms offer a compelling strategy. Lactic acid bacteria (LAB) and bifidobacteria can accumulate inorganic Se and convert it into more bioavailable organic forms, such as selenocysteine and selenomethionine. Enriching these probiotics with Se not only creates a safe and nutritious source of this essential element but may also enhance the bacteria's intrinsic functional properties, including antioxidative and anti-inflammatory activities. This approach represents a synergistic "dual-benefit" strategy for functional food design, targeting both improved Se nutrition and modulation of gut health [11]. In the realm of advanced delivery, Liu et al. presented an orally administrable, fungus-based Se microcarrier for protection against radiation-induced heart disease [12]. Advancing the frontiers of targeted therapy, Li et al. [13] developed a biomimetic platelet membrane-cloaked selenium nanoparticle (SeNP) system co-delivering a microRNA inhibitor for the precise treatment of hyperlipidemia. This system demonstrated prolonged circulation, liver-targeting capability, and dual-pathway efficacy, representing a sophisticated example of "precision nutrition" at the nanoscale.

The search for optimal Se forms and composites remains an active area of product innovation. Reviews on chitosan-based Se composites summarize how combining this biocompatible polymer with Se can enhance stability, gastrointestinal retention, and bioactivity, showcasing potential applications in functional foods and nutraceuticals [14]. Similarly, the field of selenopolysaccharides—organic compounds that combine Se with polysaccharide activities—is gaining attention. These compounds, derived from natural sources or through chemical synthesis and microbial enrichment, exhibit enhanced antioxidant, immunomodulatory, antitumor, and hypoglycemic activities compared to their separate components, offering a promising avenue for developing novel Se supplements [15].

This issue also places critical emphasis on the precision of Se status assessment and supplementation strategies. Accurate assessment of long-term Se status is fundamental. Emerging evidence suggests that biomarkers such as erythrocyte Se may provide a more reliable reflection of tissue reserves than short-term indicators like plasma Se. Equally vital is the recognition of Se's narrow therapeutic window; both deficiency and excess intake—the latter potentially inducing adverse metabolic effects such as insulin resistance—underscore the imperative for dose-specific precision in intervention strategies [16].

The research frontier continues to expand into Se's role against emerging health challenges. The protective role of Se in gastrointestinal health is further reinforced by studies utilizing advanced models. For example, research employing a gut-on-a-chip system revealed that biogenic SeNPs can ameliorate intestinal barrier oxidative damage by suppressing harmful epithelial-immune crosstalk, a finding validated in animal models [17]. Furthermore, the synthesis of highly stable, GroEL-stabilized biogenic SeNPs using probiotics has shown efficacy in alleviating experimental colitis, highlighting the potential of bio-engineered Se forms for managing inflammatory bowel diseases [18].

In summary, this Special Issue clearly illustrates that the science of Se nutrition is advancing in depth along the path of "mechanistic elucidation—product innovation—application evaluation." Future research faces both challenges and opportunities. First, achieving "form-specific precision" requires a deeper understanding of the distinct pharmacokinetics, bioavailability, and bioactivity profiles of various Se species (e.g., inorganic selenite/selenate, organic selenomethionine/selenocysteine, and SeNPs) [19]. Second, the development of natural Se-rich foods and novel Se supplements must be accompanied by robust quality and safety control systems spanning from raw materials to final prod-

https://doi.org/10.3390/nu1802032

ucts [20]. The development of stable, bio-compatible forms such as the GroEL-stabilized Bio-SeNPs points the way forward. Third, leveraging more precise biomarkers like erythrocyte Se can facilitate the transition from population-based dietary recommendations to personalized nutrition guidance based on individual status. Fourth, active exploration of Se's interventional strategies and specific applications in addressing defined health issues, such as radiation injury, environmental toxicant exposure, and metabolic syndrome, is warranted. Integrating advanced models like gut-on-a-chip into the research pipeline will further enhance the precision and human relevance of such explorations.

We sincerely thank all authors for their outstanding contributions to this Special Issue, as well as the reviewers for their expert evaluations and the editorial team for their steadfast support. We anticipate that this collection will serve not only as a compendium of current advances but also as a catalyst for future interdisciplinary research and innovation in "precision Se nutrition." Ultimately, such endeavors are vital for translating scientific evidence into effective, safe, and personalized Se strategies to improve human health globally.

Author Contributions: Resources, J.H.; writing—original draft preparation, K.Z.; writing—review and editing, J.H.; visualization, K.Z.; supervision, J.H.; project administration, J.H. All authors have read and agreed to the published version of the manuscript.

Funding: This study was supported by the 111 project from the Education Ministry of China (No. B18053).

Conflicts of Interest: The authors declare no conflicts of interest.

References

1. Rayman, M.P. Selenium and Human Health. *Lancet* **2012**, *379*, 1256–1268. [CrossRef] [PubMed]
2. Shahidin; Wang, Y.; Wu, Y.; Chen, T.; Wu, X.; Yuan, W.; Zhu, Q.; Wang, X.; Zi, C. Selenium and Selenoproteins: Mechanisms, Health Functions, and Emerging Applications. *Molecules* **2025**, *30*, 437. [CrossRef] [PubMed]
3. Bai, S.; Zhang, M.; Tang, S.; Li, M.; Wu, R.; Wan, S.; Chen, L.; Wei, X.; Feng, S. Effects and Impact of Selenium on Human Health, A Review. *Molecules* **2024**, *30*, 50. [CrossRef] [PubMed]
4. Zhang, S.; Zhang, G.; Wang, P.; Wang, L.; Fang, B.; Huang, J. Effect of Selenium and Selenoproteins on Radiation Resistance. *Nutrients* **2024**, *16*, 2902. [CrossRef]
5. Li, J.-M.; Bai, Y.-Z.; Liu, Q.-Y.; Zhang, S.-Q. Mediation Effect of Oxidative Stress on Association Between Selenium Intake and Cognition in American Adults. *Nutrients* **2024**, *16*, 4163. [CrossRef] [PubMed]
6. Huang, X.; Yang, X.; Zhang, M.; Li, T.; Zhu, K.; Dong, Y.; Lei, X.; Yu, Z.; Lv, C.; Huang, J. SELENOI Functions as a Key Modulator of Ferroptosis Pathway in Colitis and Colorectal Cancer. *Adv. Sci.* **2024**, *11*, 2404073. [CrossRef] [PubMed]
7. Zhang, X.; Xiong, W.; Chen, L.-L.; Huang, J.-Q.; Lei, X.G. Selenoprotein V Protects against Endoplasmic Reticulum Stress and Oxidative Injury Induced by Pro-Oxidants. *Free Radic. Biol. Med.* **2020**, *160*, 670–679. [CrossRef] [PubMed]
8. Chen, L.-L.; Huang, J.-Q.; Wu, Y.-Y.; Chen, L.-B.; Li, S.-P.; Zhang, X.; Wu, S.; Ren, F.-Z.; Lei, X.-G. Loss of Selenov Predisposes Mice to Extra Fat Accumulation and Attenuated Energy Expenditure. *Redox Biol.* **2021**, *45*, 102048. [CrossRef] [PubMed]
9. Zhu, J.; Lv, Q.; Li, F.; Xu, P.; Han, Z.; Yang, A.; Shi, Z.; Wang, C.; Jiang, J.; Zhu, Y.; et al. Alleviation of Lipid Disorder and Liver Damage in High-Fat Diet-Induced Obese Mice by Selenium-Enriched Cardamine Violifolia with Cadmium Accumulation. *Nutrients* **2024**, *16*, 3208. [CrossRef] [PubMed]
10. Li, H.; Liu, H.; Tang, X.; Deng, Z.; Li, H. From Soil to Table: A Comprehensive Review of Selenium-Fortified Foods. *Compr. Rev. Food Sci. Food Saf.* **2025**, *24*, e70250. [CrossRef] [PubMed]
11. Pophaly, S.D.; Poonam; Singh, P.; Kumar, H.; Tomar, S.K.; Singh, R. Selenium Enrichment of Lactic Acid Bacteria and Bifidobacteria: A Functional Food Perspective. *Trends Food Sci. Technol.* **2014**, *39*, 135–145. [CrossRef]
12. Liu, C.; Wang, W.; Lai, H.; Chen, Y.; Li, L.; Li, H.; Zhan, M.; Chen, T.; Cao, W.; Li, X. Biosynthesis of Fungus-Based Oral Selenium Microcarriers for Radioprotection and Immuno-Homeostasis Shaping against Radiation-Induced Heart Disease. *Bioact. Mater.* **2024**, *37*, 393–406. [CrossRef] [PubMed]
13. Li, T.; Liu, L.; Zhu, K.; Luo, Y.; Huang, X.; Dong, Y.; Huang, J. Biomimetic MicroRNAs-Selenium-Nanocomposites for Targeted and Combined Hyperlipidemia Therapy. *Adv. Heal. Mater.* **2024**, *13*, e2400064. [CrossRef] [PubMed]
14. Chen, W.; Li, X.; Cheng, H.; Xia, W. Chitosan-Based Selenium Composites as Potent Se Supplements: Synthesis, Beneficial Health Effects, and Applications in Food and Agriculture. *Trends Food Sci. Technol.* **2022**, *129*, 339–352. [CrossRef]

https://doi.org/10.3390/nu18020320

15. Yang, W.; Huang, G.; Chen, F.; Huang, H. Extraction/Synthesis and Biological Activities of Selenopolysaccharide. *Trends Food Sci. Technol.* **2021**, *109*, 211–218. [CrossRef]
16. Rayman, M.P. Selenium Intake, Status, and Health: A Complex Relationship. *Hormones* **2020**, *19*, 9–14. [CrossRef] [PubMed]
17. Qiao, L.; Yang, G.; Deng, T.; Chang, J.; Dou, X.; Song, X.; Zeng, X.; Ren, L.; Xu, C. Prophylactic Supplementation with Biogenic Selenium Nanoparticles Mitigated Intestinal Barrier Oxidative Damage through Suppressing Epithelial-Immune Crosstalk with Gut-on-a-Chip. *J. Adv. Res.* **2025**. [CrossRef] [PubMed]
18. Li, T.; Zhu, K.; Wang, L.; Dong, Y.; Huang, J. Stabilization by Chaperone GroEL in Biogenic Selenium Nanoparticles Produced from Bifidobacterium Animalis H15 for the Treatment of DSS-Induced Colitis. *ACS Appl. Mater. Interfaces* **2024**, *16*, 13439–13452. [CrossRef] [PubMed]
19. Hou, X.; Wang, Z.; Peng, M. Selenium Compounds and Their Bioactivities: Molecular Mechanisms and Prospects for Functional Food and Therapeutic Applications. *Plants* **2025**, *14*, 2622. [CrossRef] [PubMed]
20. Chen, N.; Zhao, C.; Zhang, T. Selenium Transformation and Selenium-Rich Foods. *Food Biosci.* **2021**, *40*, 100875. [CrossRef]

https://doi.org/10.3390/nu18020320

nutrients

MDPI

Article

Dietary Fatty Acids and Antinuclear Antibodies Among Adults with Arthritis in the United States: NHANES 1999–2004

Jie Guo [1,†], Yifei Yu [1,†], Jiaqi Su [2,†], Fazheng Ren [1] and Juan Chen [1,*]

1 Department of Nutrition and Health, Key Laboratory of Precision Nutrition and Food Quality, China Agricultural University, Beijing 100091, China; guojie@cau.edu.cn (J.G.)
2 Department of Health Sciences and Technology, ETH Zurich, 8092 Zurich, Switzerland
* Correspondence: chenjuan@cau.edu.cn
† These authors contributed equally to this work.

Abstract: Background: This study investigated the link between daily fatty acid intake and antinuclear antibody (ANA) levels, a marker of immune dysregulation and autoimmune diseases, in individuals with self-reported arthritis. **Methods**: From the US National Health and Nutrition Examination Survey (NHANES) 1999–2004, 829 participants who self-reported arthritis and had autoantibody measurements were selected. Dietary fatty acids were collected via two 24 h dietary recall interviews conducted by trained interviewers. ANA levels were collected by measuring IgG autoantibodies targeting cellular antigens. **Results**: In a multi-adjusted logistic model, the odds ratio (OR) of the highest tertile of omega-3 intake (with omega-3 intake > 1.60 g/day) for the probability of ANA positivity was 0.43 (95% CI: 0.19–0.96) compared to those in the lowest tertile (≤0.92 g/day). However, we did not observe statistically significant results for other fatty acids. **Conclusions**: Our findings highlight the potential of dietary omega-3 PUFAs to modulate immune function and lower the risk of ANA positivity in individuals with arthritis.

Keywords: arthritis; dietary fatty acid; omega-3 PUFAs; antinuclear antibodies; NHANES

1. Introduction

Immune-inflammatory diseases represent a diverse spectrum of disorders characterized by chronic inflammation, immune system dysregulation, and tissue damage. Among these, arthritis encompasses a group of debilitating conditions including rheumatoid arthritis and osteoarthritis, which significantly impact quality of life [1,2]. Arthritis manifests as persistent joint pain, swelling, and progressive cartilage destruction, ultimately resulting in reduced physical function and a substantial socioeconomic burden. The pathophysiology of arthritis arises from a complex interplay of genetic, environmental, and lifestyle factors. Notably, diet has emerged as a modifiable factor influencing disease progression and symptom management [3].

Dietary fatty acids, particularly polyunsaturated fatty acids (PUFAs), have garnered considerable attention for their immunomodulatory and anti-inflammatory effects [4–6]. Previous research has highlighted the role of omega-3 PUFAs, such as eicosapentaenoic acid (EPA) and docosahexaenoic acid (DHA), in mitigating inflammatory responses by modulating cytokine production, reducing oxidative stress, and promoting the resolution of inflammation [7–9]. Conversely, omega-6 fatty acids, while generally associated with pro-inflammatory effects, may exhibit more nuanced effects depending on their balance with omega-3 fatty acids [10,11]. Observational and interventional studies have consistently reported the association between increased dietary intake or supplementation of specific fatty acids and improvements in arthritis symptoms, including a reduction in joint pain, stiffness, and systemic inflammation [12]. However, despite these promising findings, the impact of broader fatty acid profiles on arthritis, particularly their interplay with immune markers, remains insufficiently underexplored.

Antinuclear antibodies (ANAs) are autoantibodies targeting nuclear components of cells and serve as hallmark biomarkers for systemic autoimmune diseases, including systemic lupus erythematosus and rheumatoid arthritis [13–15]. The presence of ANAs indicates dysregulation of immune tolerance and heightened autoimmune activity, making them critical diagnostic and prognostic indicators for arthritis-related conditions [16]. Beyond their diagnostic role, ANAs may contribute to disease pathogenesis by forming immune complexes that exacerbate inflammation and tissue damage [17,18]. Their prevalence varies among populations, with significant implications for identifying individuals at risk of developing arthritis or monitoring disease activity. Understanding the factors that influence ANA levels, including dietary components, is therefore crucial for elucidating the complex interactions between nutrition, immunity, and arthritis.

We hypothesized that it is possible for ANA levels to correlate with different types of fatty acids in the population. This study investigates the link between daily intake of 19 fatty acids and ANA presence in US adults with arthritis, using NHANES 1999–2004 data. It aims to provide insights into dietary strategies for modulating immune responses and slowing arthritis progression.

2. Materials and Methods

The National Health and Nutrition Examination Survey, a program by the Centers for Disease Control and Prevention in collaboration with the National Center for Health Statistics, assesses the health and nutrition of the U.S. population living outside of institutions. Using a stratified multistage probability sampling method, NHANES collects comprehensive data through household interviews, physical examinations at mobile examination centers, and laboratory analyses of biological specimens. To ensure adequate representation of key demographic subgroups, such as racial and ethnic minorities, children, and older adults, the survey incorporates an oversampling strategy. NHANES operates as a continuous program, with data released in biennial cycles. Study protocols are reviewed and approved by an Institutional Review Board, with informed consent obtained from all participants [19].

2.1. Study Population

The study utilized data collected from the NHANES 1999–2004, focusing on individuals who self-reported arthritis. Initially, a cohort of 3978 participants with self-reported arthritis was identified. To minimize potential confounding, we further excluded pregnant and lactating women (n = 42), participants without autoantibody measurements (n = 3071), and participants without dietary fatty acid intake information (n = 36). After these exclusions, the final analytical cohort comprised 829 participants with self-reported arthritis, and complete autoantibody measurements and dietary fatty acid intake data were included in the analysis (Figure 1).

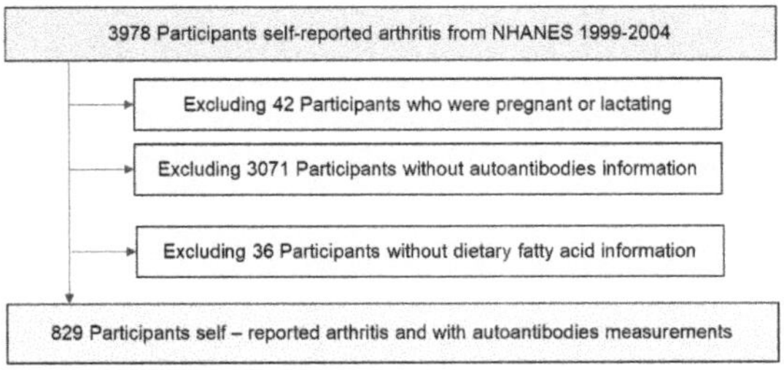

Figure 1. Flow chart of the study population.

2.2. Assessment of Dietary Fatty Acids

Dietary fatty acids were estimated using data from one (1999–2000 and 2001–2002) or two (2003–2004) 24 h dietary recall interviews. Since cycle 2003–2004, the dietary recall interviews have been conducted twice for each participant: The first interview was conducted at the Mobile Examination Center, followed by a second interview via phone, 3 to 10 days later. Nutrient and micronutrient intake were assessed using data from the U.S. Department of Agriculture database, while saturated fatty acid (SFA), monounsaturated fatty acid (MUFA), polyunsaturated fatty acid (PUFA), and decanoic acid were derived from the NHANES 1999–2004 database directly. Moreover, omega-3 PUFA (ω-3 PUFA) was calculated by summing the intake of alpha-linolenic acid, stearic acid, eicosapentaenoic acid, docosapentenoic acid, and docosahexaenoic acid. Omega-6 PUFA (ω-6 PUFA) was calculated by summing the intake of linoleic acid and arachidonic acid. The decanoic acid to ω-3 PUFA ratio and ω-3 to ω-6 ratio were calculated. To facilitate analysis, the dietary intakes of these fatty acids, and the ratios between them, were then categorized into tertiles for further analysis [20–22].

2.3. Assessment of ANA Test

ANA titers were determined using stored serum samples from a one-third subsample of NHANES participants aged 12 years and older. ANA screening was conducted using the indirect immunofluorescence assay on HEp-2 cells [23]. IgG autoantibodies targeting cellular antigens were detected, and fluorescence staining intensity was graded on a scale from 0 to 4. Samples with a staining intensity ≥ 3 are defined as ANA positive, and samples with a staining intensity of less than 3 are ANA negative. The cellular staining patterns, such as speckled, nucleolar, and homogeneous, were assessed according to their anatomical distribution of intracellular antigens and recorded using a reference gallery. This approach, combining immunofluorescence and immunoprecipitation, ensured precise identification of ANA titers and specificities, providing a reliable estimate of autoantibody prevalence and characteristics within the U.S. population during the study period [24,25].

2.4. Covariates

To account for potential confounding factors, relevant demographic and socioeconomic information was obtained from the NHANES study to account for potential covariates. In the multi-adjusted model, we included age, sex, race/ethnicity (non-Hispanic White, non-Hispanic Black, Mexican American, and other Hispanic or other race), highest education level (less than high school, high school or equivalent, college or above), smoking status (current, former, never), alcohol consumption status (non-drinker, drinker), marital status (married or living with a partner, not married nor living with a partner), and poverty-to-income ratio (categorized as <1.3, 1.3–3.5, and $\geq$3.5). These variables were selected due to their potential confounding effect for the association between fatty acids and ANA level [26,27].

2.5. Statistical Analysis

The 6-year survey weights extracted from the ANA database were systematically applied across all analyses to appropriately adjust for NHANES's complex sampling design. Baseline characteristics were described as weighted means and standard errors or percentages among total, ANA-negative, and ANA-positive participants.

Logistic regression models were applied to examine the odds ratio (OR) and 95% confidence interval (CI) for the relationship between ANA status and dietary fatty acids, categorized into tertiles, with the lowest tertile serving as the reference group. In the logistic regression models, we first controlled for age, sex, and race/ethnicity (Model 1), then made further adjustments for education level, marital status, and poverty-to-income ratio (Model 2), and subsequently adjusted for drinking status, smoking status, and total energy intake (Model 3). We further explored the ORs of continuous dietary fatty acid with ANA status using the restricted cubic spline with four knots at the 5th, 35th, 65th, and 95th percentiles.

Statistical analyses were conducted with SAS 9.4, employing two-tailed tests with a significance threshold of $p < 0.05$. Weighted estimates, including proportions and means (±SE), were generated through the SURVEYFREQ and SURVEYMEANS procedures. Multiple comparison adjustments were implemented using the Bonferroni method. The SURVEYLOGISTIC procedure was used to calculate the OR (95% CI). Data were analyzed from November 2024 to January 2025.

2.6. Ethical Approval and Consent to Participate

All analyses were conducted using publicly available databases. The Institutional Review Board for the National Center for Health Statistics approved the NHANES, which was performed in accordance with the Declaration of Helsinki. All participants provided written informed consent before data collection.

3. Results

3.1. Baseline Characteristics

Table 1 presents the baseline characteristics of the study population stratified by ANA status. The mean age of participants was 59.8 (standard deviation: 0.6) years and 60.9% were females. Participants who were ANA positive were more likely to be females, to never have been smokers, and to have lower levels of omega 3 PUFAs, omega 6 PUFAs, MUFAs, and PUFAs.

Table 1. Baseline characteristics of study population by ANA status (N = 865).

Characteristics	Total	ANA Positive	ANA Negative	*p*-Value
Age, mean (SD), years	59.8 (0.6)	62.4 (1.5)	59.3 (0.6)	0.099
Sex (%)				0.018
Female	492 (60.9)	88 (70.1)	404 (59.2)	
Male	337 (39.1)	46 (29.9)	291 (40.8)	
Race/Ethnicity (%)				0.530
Mexican American	142 (3.6)	19 (3.3)	123 (3.6)	
Non-Hispanic White	490 (77.1)	76 (73.6)	414 (77.8)	
Non-Hispanic Black	147 (11.4)	29 (14.9)	118 (10.7)	
Other Hispanic or other race	50 (7.9)	10 (8.2)	40 (7.9)	
Married status (%)				0.178
Married or living with a partner	472 (63.2)	68 (56.6)	404 (64.4)	
Not married nor living with a partner	332 (36.8)	63 (43.4)	269 (35.6)	

Table 1. *Cont.*

Characteristics	Total	ANA Positive	ANA Negative	p-Value
Poverty-to-income ratio (%)				0.485
<1.3	240 (24.2)	34 (20.2)	206 (24.9)	
1.3–3.5	313 (40.2)	54 (45.8)	259 (39.2)	
≥3.5	211 (35.6)	33 (34.0)	178 (35.9)	
Highest education (%)				0.859
Less than high school	319 (27.2)	49 (26.8)	270 (27.3)	
High school or equivalent	193 (27.5)	33 (29.6)	160 (27.1)	
College or above	315 (45.3)	52 (43.7)	263 (45.6)	
Smoking status (%)				<0.001
Current	162 (20.8)	17 (11.6)	145 (22.5)	
Former	302 (36.3)	45 (30.4)	257 (37.4)	
Never	365 (42.9)	72 (58.0)	293 (40.1)	
Drinking status (%)				0.242
Non-drinker	296 (34.7)	41 (28.9)	255 (35.7)	
Drinker	505 (65.3)	85 (71.1)	420 (64.3)	
Total energy, mean (SD), kcal	1987 (42.5)	1874.9 (78.5)	2008.9 (48.6)	0.182
Omega 3 PUFAs, mean (SD), g	1.6 (0.0)	1.4 (0.1)	1.6 (0.1)	0.031
Decanoic (g)	0.4 (0.0)	0.4 (0.0)	0.4 (0.0)	0.620
Decanoic: omega 3 PUFAs ratio	0.3 (0.0)	0.3 (0.0)	0.3 (0.0)	0.501
Omega 6 PUFAs (g)	14.4 (0.4)	12.7 (0.6)	14.7 (0.4)	0.014
Omega 3: omega 6 PUFAs ratio	0.1 (0.0)	0.1 (0.0)	0.1 (0.0)	0.021
SFAs (g)	25.1 (0.7)	23.2 (1.3)	25.5 (0.8)	0.170
MUFAs (g)	28.5 (0.8)	25.7 (1.3)	29.1 (0.9)	0.045
PUFAs (g)	16.2 (0.4)	14.3 (0.7)	16.5 (0.5)	0.016

Abbreviations: ANA, antinuclear antibody; SFA, saturated fatty acid; MUFA, monounsaturated fatty acid; PUFA, polyunsaturated fatty acid. Data are presented as weighted means (standard error) for continuous variables and weighted percentages for categorical variables.

3.2. Associations of Dietary Fatty Acids Intake with the Probability of Being ANA Positive

Table 2 presents the ORs and 95% CIs for the association between various dietary fatty acids and ANA positivity. In Model 1, the OR (95% CI) of the highest tertile of omega-3 intake (with omega-3 intake > 1.60 g/day) for the probability of being ANA positive was 0.62 (95% CI: 0.40–0.96) compared to those in the lowest tertile (≤0.92 g/day), which was still statistically significant after multi-adjustment (0.43 [95% CI: 0.19–0.96]). However, other fatty acids such as decanoic acid, omega-6 PUFAs, SFAs, MUFAs, and total PUFAs did not demonstrate any significant associations with ANA positivity.

The associations between dietary intake of 19 fatty acids and the probability of ANA positivity were explored, and the results reveal that only omega-3 polyunsaturated fatty acids have a significant protective effect against ANA positivity. Individuals in the highest tertile of omega-3 intake (>1.60 g/day) exhibited a substantially reduced likelihood of ANA positivity compared to those in the lowest tertile (≤0.92 g/day). In Model 3, the OR for ANA positivity in the highest tertile was 0.43 (95% CI: 0.19–0.96), suggesting that higher omega-3 consumption is associated with a significantly lower risk of ANA positivity. These findings highlight the unique and beneficial role of omega-3 fatty acids in reducing the risk of ANA positivity, potentially through their anti-inflammatory and immunomodulatory properties. However, other dietary fatty acids appear to have no significant impact on ANA status (Figure 2).

Table 2. Odds ratios and 95% confidence intervals of dietary fatty acid intake for ANA positivity.

Dietary Fatty Acid	Model 1	Model 2	Model 3
Decanoic (g)			
Tertile 1 (≤0.17)	Reference	Reference	Reference
Tertile 2 (>0.17, ≤0.42)	0.66 (0.36–1.21)	0.59 (0.31–1.16)	0.58 (0.28–1.21)
Tertile 3 (>0.42)	0.99 (0.54–1.83)	0.98 (0.51–1.86)	0.97 (0.45–2.08)
Omega-3 (g)			
Tertile 1 (≤0.92)	Reference	Reference	Reference
Tertile 2 (>0.92, ≤1.60)	0.67 (0.41–1.11)	0.65 (0.38–1.13)	0.59 (0.30–1.17)
Tertile 3 (>1.60)	0.62 (0.40–0.96)	0.55 (0.35–0.86)	0.43 (0.19–0.96)
Decanoic: omega 3 PUFAs ratio			
Tertile 1 (≤0.14)	Reference	Reference	Reference
Tertile 2 (>0.14, ≤0.33)	1.20 (0.74–1.95)	1.16 (0.73–1.84)	1.14 (0.73–1.78)
Tertile 3 (>0.33)	1.57 (0.78–3.17)	1.70 (0.81–3.58)	1.64 (0.75–3.60)
Omega-6 (g)			
Tertile 1 (≤8.79)	Reference	Reference	Reference
Tertile 2 (>8.79, ≤15.13)	1.03 (0.67–1.59)	1.01 (0.63–1.64)	1.04 (0.57–1.89)
Tertile 3 (>15.13)	0.87 (0.52–1.45)	0.89 (0.51–1.53)	0.82 (0.36–1.85)
Omega 3: omega 6 PUFAs ratio			
Tertile 1 (≤0.09)	Reference	Reference	Reference
Tertile 2 (>0.09, ≤0.12)	1.21 (0.76–1.94)	1.11 (0.70–1.74)	1.22 (0.75–1.98)
Tertile 3 (>0.12)	0.78 (0.49–1.25)	0.66 (0.43–1.03)	0.71 (0.45–1.13)
SFAs (g)			
Tertile 1 (≤15.75)	Reference	Reference	Reference
Tertile 2 (>15.75, ≤25.41)	0.98 (0.60–1.62)	0.92 (0.57–1.49)	0.97 (0.53–1.78)
Tertile 3 (>25.41)	0.98 (0.55–1.75)	0.97 (0.55–1.72)	1.07 (0.41–2.75)
MUFAs (g)			
Tertile 1 (≤17.89)	Reference	Reference	Reference
Tertile 2 (>17.89, ≤29.67)	1.14 (0.68–1.91)	1.31 (0.82–2.09)	1.38 (0.81–2.35)
Tertile 3 (>29.67)	0.86 (0.48–1.56)	0.90 (0.49–1.67)	0.93 (0.40–2.20)
PUFAs (g)			
Tertile 1 (≤9.90)	Reference	Reference	Reference
Tertile 2 (>9.90, ≤17.15)	1.01 (0.64–1.59)	1.00 (0.60–1.67)	1.01 (0.53–1.91)
Tertile 3 (>17.15)	0.85 (0.52–1.41)	0.86 (0.51–1.45)	0.75 (0.34–1.68)

Abbreviations: ANA, antinuclear antibody; SFA, saturated fatty acid; MUFA, monounsaturated fatty acid; PUFA, polyunsaturated fatty acid. Model 1 adjusted for age, sex, and race/ethnicity. Model 2 further adjusted for education level, marital status, and poverty-to-income ratio. Model 3 further adjusted for drinking status, smoking status, and total energy intake.

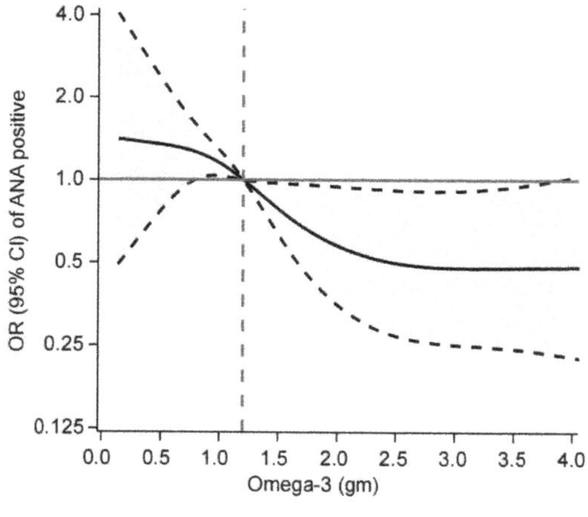

Figure 2. OR (95% CI) of ANA positivity in relation to dietary omega-3 intake.

The odds ratio (OR) and 95% confidence interval (CI) were calculated using multivariable logistic regression models with restricted cubic splines. The model was adjusted for age, sex, race/ethnicity, education level, marital status, poverty-to-income ratio, drinking status, smoking status, and total energy intake. The *p*-value for overall association and *p*-value for linear association were both <0.05.

4. Discussion

Our study explored the relationships between ANA positivity and 19 dietary fatty acids, including omega-3 and omega-6 polyunsaturated fatty acids, as well as monounsaturated and saturated fatty acids. The most significant finding was a strong inverse association between dietary omega-3 PUFA intake and the probability of ANA positivity. Participants in the highest tertile of omega-3 intake (>1.60 g/day) demonstrated a 57% reduced likelihood of ANA positivity compared to those in the lowest tertile ($\leq$0.92 g/day), with the relationship remaining robust across multiple adjustment models. In contrast, none of the other dietary fatty acids, including omega-6 PUFAs, SFAs, MUFAs, or their ratios, exhibited statistically significant associations with ANA positivity. These findings underscore the role of omega-3 PUFAs in modulating immune function and potentially mitigating autoimmune risk.

The inverse association between omega-3 intake and ANA positivity aligns with prior research demonstrating the anti-inflammatory and immunomodulatory effects of omega-3 PUFAs. For example, research consistently shows that omega-3 fatty acids, especially EPA and DHA, are linked to lower levels of pro-inflammatory cytokines like TNF-α, IL-1β, and IL-6 [28–30]. These cytokines play critical roles in the pathogenesis of autoimmune diseases. Furthermore, omega-3 fatty acid supplementation has demonstrated reductions in disease activity and symptom severity in autoimmune diseases such as rheumatoid arthritis [31], lupus [32], and multiple sclerosis [33]. While direct studies linking omega-3 PUFA intake to ANA positivity are limited, the observed protective effects are consistent with their role in immune regulation. Notably, this study did not find significant associations between omega-6 PUFAs and ANA positivity. This result is consistent with mixed evidence regarding omega-6 fatty acids and inflammation [34]. Omega-6 PUFAs have a complex relationship with inflammation. While they are precursors to pro-inflammatory eicosanoids (e.g., prostaglandins and leukotrienes), they also contribute to the generation of anti-inflammatory mediators under certain conditions [35,36]. The balance between omega-6 and omega-3 fatty acids intake is crucial for maintaining immune homeostasis, and prior studies have suggested that an increased ratio of omega-6 to omega-3 intake may exacerbate inflammatory processes [35,37]. However, no significant effects of this ratio on ANA positivity were observed, potentially due to the relatively low omega-6 intake in the study population or unaccounted for confounders. Current direct studies directly examining the relationship between dietary fatty acids and ANA positivity remain limited. However the prevalence of ANA has been explored in the context of other inflammatory and autoimmune diseases. For example, in Hispanic children with NAFLD, ANA positivity was associated with insulin resistance and lower levels of HDL cholesterol levels [38]. Additionally, serum linoleic acid concentrations were found to correlate positively with ANA titers in SLE patients [39].

The observed protective effect of omega-3 PUFAs on ANA positivity may be mediated by several interconnected mechanisms. Based on previous literature studies, omega-3 PUFAs are well-documented modulators of inflammatory pathways. They are integrated into cell membranes, where they compete with omega-6 PUFAs for cyclooxygenase and lipoxygenase enzyme substrates. This leads to a shift in eicosanoid profiles, favoring less pro-inflammatory and more anti-inflammatory eicosanoids [40,41]. This shift in eicosanoid profiles may reduce systemic inflammation and autoantibody production, both of which are critical contributors to ANA positivity and the pathogenesis of autoimmune diseases. Beyond these, omega-3 PUFAs may further reduce ANA levels by altering lipid raft dynamics in immune cell membranes. Importantly, omega-3 PUFAs are associated with downregulation of the nuclear factor κB (NFκB) signaling pathway, which is a master switch regulating the expression of many pro-inflammatory genes. Omega-3 PUFAs inhibit NF-κB/MAPK signaling, thereby inhibiting autoreactive B cell activation and nuclear antigen exposure [42,43]. Omega-3 PUFAs also modulate immune cell function. They can reduce the activation of pro-inflammatory M1 macrophages and enhance the differentiation of anti-inflammatory M2 macrophages [44–46]. Similarly, omega-3 PUFAs inhibit the activation of Th17 cells, a subset of the T-helpers cell subset implicated in autoimmunity, while enhancing the activity of regulatory T cells, which support immune tolerance [44]. These immunomodulatory effects could directly impact ANA production and the development of autoimmune conditions. Furthermore, omega-3 PUFAs may exert their effects through epigenetic modifications [47]. Emerging evidence suggests that omega-3 fatty acids can alter DNA methylation, histone acetylation, and microRNA expression, leading to changes in gene expression patterns involved in inflammation and immunity [48,49]. These epigenetic effects could provide a mechanistic link between dietary omega-3 intake and reduced ANA positivity. Metabolically, EPA acts as an endogenous PPARγ ligand to reprogram dendritic cell metabolism toward fatty acid oxidation, inhibiting mTORC1-mediated cytokine release and enhancing Nrf2 activity to reduce ROS-induced DNA damage and neutrophil extracellular trap formation, thereby limiting modified nuclear antigen generation [50]. Moreover, the gut microbiota may serve as a mediator of the protective effects of omega-3 fatty acids. Omega-3 PUFAs are known to alter gut microbiota composition, enhancing the abundance of beneficial bacteria like Bifidobacterium and Lactobacillus while decreasing pro-inflammatory taxa [51,52]. Healthy gut microbiota can strengthen the intestinal barrier, reduce systemic inflammation, and enhance immune regulation, all of which may contribute to lower ANA positivity.

A strength of this study is that we used a nationally representative sample of the U.S. population for the analyses, with various dietary fatty acids and ANA assessed following standardized procedures. Nevertheless, some limitations need to be acknowledged. First, dietary data were collected based on self-reported 24 h dietary recalls, which are subject to recall bias and may not accurately represent habitual intake. Considering that people tend to think in a positive way, they will overestimate their fatty acid intake and may be wrongly classified, which will lead to an underestimation of our results. The reliance on a single or limited number of dietary recalls may also fail to capture long-term dietary patterns. Second, the form of consumption of unsaturated fatty acids and the duration of consumption may also matter. However, we could not consider these factors because they were not collected in the NHANES. Further studies with more detailed information are warranted to comprehensively assess the association between fatty acids and ANA levels. Third, we could not conclude the causal association due to the cross-sectional study design. Further studies using longitudinal data are needed to confirm these findings and elucidate causality. Then, the sample size of ANA-positive individuals was relatively small, which may limit the generalizability of our results. To validate our findings and investigate potential interactions between dietary fatty acids and other demographic or lifestyle factors, larger studies with more diverse populations are needed. Finally, the data used in this study were derived from the NHANES 1999–2004 cycles, and dietary patterns may have shifted since then. Future studies should examine more recent datasets to determine whether these associations persist in contemporary populations.

5. Conclusions

This study provides novel evidence associating higher dietary omega-3 PUFA intake with a reduced likelihood of ANA positivity in individuals with arthritis. These finding suggesting a potential role for omega-3 fatty acids in modulating immune function and lowering autoimmune risk. These results highlight the importance of dietary interventions as a strategy for preventing and managing immune-related conditions. In addition, further studies, such as animal experiments and randomized clinical trials, are warranted to elaborate the underlying mechanisms of the protective effect of omega-3 PUFAs on autoimmune diseases and to explore the therapeutic effect of omega-3 PUFAs on autoimmune diseases in the population. Further research is warranted to confirm these results, elucidate the underlying biological mechanisms, and examine the broader implications of omega-3 fatty acid intake in the context of autoimmune disease contexts.

Author Contributions: Conceptualization, J.G. and Y.Y.; methodology, J.G. and J.C.; software, J.G.; validation, J.G., Y.Y., J.S. and J.C.; formal analysis, J.G.; investigation, J.G., Y.Y. and J.S.; resources, F.R. and J.C.; data curation, J.G.; writing—original draft preparation, J.G., Y.Y. and J.S.; writing—review and editing, J.G., Y.Y., J.S., F.R. and J.C.; visualization, J.G.; supervision, F.R. and J.C.; project administration, J.C.; funding acquisition, J.C. All authors have read and agreed to the published version of the manuscript.

Funding: This research was funded by the National Key Research and Development Program of China, grant number 2023YFF1103503 (to Juan Chen).

Institutional Review Board Statement: Ethical review and approval were waived for this study because it utilizes publicly available NHANES data that has already been reviewed and approved by the Institutional Review Board.

Informed Consent Statement: Patient consent was waived as it uses publicly available NHANES data, where all participants had already provided written informed consent.

Data Availability Statement: All relevant data in this study are publicly available on the National Health and Nutrition Examination Survey Homepage (https://www.cdc.gov/nchs/nhanes/index.html (accessed on 4 March 2025)). The corresponding author Dr Juan Chen (email address: chenjuan@cau.edu.cn) should be contacted for any requests (e.g., data used for all analyses; analytic code; any other materials used in the current study).

Conflicts of Interest: The authors declare no conflicts of interest. The funders had no role in the analyses and interpretation of data.

Abbreviations

The following abbreviations are used in this manuscript:

ANA	antinuclear antibodies
CI	confidence interval
DHA	docosahexaenoic acid
EPA	eicosapentaenoic acid
MUFA	monounsaturated fatty acid
NHANES	National Health and Nutrition Examination Survey
OR	odds ratio
PUFA	polyunsaturated fatty acid
SFA	saturated fatty acid

References

1. Wang, F.F.; Liu, J.; Fang, Y.Y.; Wen, J.T.; He, M.Y.; Li, X.; Han, Q. Effect of *Siegesbeckiae Herba* on immune-inflammation of rheumatoid arthritis: Data mining and network pharmacology. *Eur. J. Integr. Med.* **2023**, *59*, 102242. [CrossRef]
2. Chen, W.J.; Sun, Z.; Xiong, X.H.; Tan, H.T.; Hu, J.H.; Liu, C.R.; Chen, C. Exploring the causal link among statin drugs and the osteoarthritis risk based on Mendelian randomization research. *Front. Genet.* **2024**, *15*, 1390387. [CrossRef] [PubMed]
3. Akey, K.S.; Esakkimuthukumar, M.; Saranya, R.; Chandru, M.; Sowbarnika, S.; Sudharsan, J.; Dhanush, V.; Prabha, T.; Jubie, S. Exploring Potential Bioactive Components of Persea americana for the Treatment of Rheumatoid Arthritis through Network Pharmacology. *Curr. Rheumatol. Rev.* **2024**, *in press*. [CrossRef] [PubMed]
4. Stándo, M.; Piatek, P.; Namiecinska, M.; Lewkowicz, P.; Lewkowicz, N. Omega-3 Polyunsaturated Fatty Acids EPA and DHA as an Adjunct to Non-Surgical Treatment of Periodontitis: A Randomized Clinical Trial. *Nutrients* **2020**, *12*, 2614. [CrossRef]
5. Laing, B.B.; Cavadino, A.; Ellett, S.; Ferguson, L.R. Effects of an Omega-3 and Vitamin D Supplement on Fatty Acids and Vitamin D Serum Levels in Double-Blinded, Randomized, Controlled Trials in Healthy and Crohn's Disease Populations. *Nutrients* **2020**, *12*, 1139. [CrossRef]
6. Pisaniello, A.D.; Psaltis, P.J.; King, P.M.; Liu, G.; Gibson, R.A.; Tan, J.T.; Duong, M.; Nguyen, T.; Bursill, C.A.; Worthley, M.I.; et al. Omega-3 fatty acids ameliorate vascular inflammation: A rationale for their atheroprotective effects. *Atherosclerosis* **2021**, *324*, 27–37. [CrossRef]
7. Xu, Y.; Zhang, H.; Yang, H.T.; Liu, C.D.; Song, C.Y.; Cheng, Y.Y.; He, C.; Zou, Z.; Zhou, D.; Wu, G.; et al. Eicosapentaenoic acid and docosahexaenoic acid suppress colonic tumorigenesis in obese mice. *J. Funct. Foods* **2024**, *116*, 106164. [CrossRef]
8. Tan, W.F.; Mao, L.Z.; Yu, S.Y.; Huang, J.; Xie, Q.Y.; Hu, M.J.; Mao, L. DHA and EPA improve liver IR in HFD-induced IR mice through modulating the gut microbiotas-LPS-liver axis. *J. Funct. Foods* **2024**, *112*, 105917. [CrossRef]
9. Dawczynski, C.; Dittrich, M.; Neumann, T.; Goetze, K.; Welzel, A.; Oelzner, P.; Völker, S.; Schaible, A.; Troisi, F.; Thomas, L.; et al. Docosahexaenoic acid in the treatment of rheumatoid arthritis: A double-blind, placebo-controlled, randomized cross-over study with microalgae vs. sunflower oil. *Clin. Nutr.* **2018**, *37*, 494–504. [CrossRef]
10. Jeong, H.Y.; Moon, Y.S.; Cho, K.K. ω-6 and ω-3 Polyunsaturated Fatty Acids: Inflammation, Obesity and Foods of Animal Resources. *Food Sci. Anim. Resour.* **2024**, *44*, 988–1010. [CrossRef]
11. Yan, D.; Ye, S.Y.; He, Y.; Wang, S.D.; Xiao, Y.; Xiang, X.; Deng, M.; Luo, W.; Chen, X.; Wang, X. Fatty acids and lipid mediators in inflammatory bowel disease: From mechanism to treatment. *Front. Immunol.* **2023**, *14*, 1286667. [CrossRef] [PubMed]
12. Caballero-Solares, A.; Eslamloo, K.; Hall, J.R.; Katan, T.; Emam, M.; Xue, X.; Taylor, R.G.; Balder, R.; Parrish, C.C.; Rise, M.L. Vegetable omega-3 and omega-6 fatty acids differentially modulate the antiviral and antibacterial immune responses of Atlantic salmon. *Sci. Rep.* **2024**, *14*, 10947. [CrossRef] [PubMed]
13. Pisetsky, D.S.; Spencer, D.M.; Rovin, B.; Lipsky, P.E. Role of ANA testing in the classification of patients with systemic lupus erythematosus. *Ann. Rheum. Dis.* **2021**, *80*, e124. [CrossRef] [PubMed]
14. Kondeti, R.D.; Venkatesh, K.; Murthy, D.; Kameti, S.; Devi, K.S.; Chandrika, K.V. A Study of Clinical Manifestations and their Association with Antinuclear Antibodies in Various Autoimmune Connective Tissue Disorders. *Indian J. Dermatol.* **2023**, *68*, 486. [CrossRef]
15. Andrade, L.E.C.; Damoiseaux, J.; Vergani, D.; Fritzler, M.J. Antinuclear antibodies (ANA) as a criterion for classification and diagnosis of systemic autoimmune diseases. *J. Transl. Autoimmun.* **2022**, *5*, 100145. [CrossRef]
16. Nanda, R.; Gupta, P.; Patel, S.; Shah, S.; Mohapatra, E. Uncommon antinuclear antibody patterns as diagnostic indicators. *Clin. Biochem.* **2021**, *90*, 28–33. [CrossRef]
17. Kuwana, M.; Gil-Vila, A.; Selva-O'Callaghan, A. Role of autoantibodies in the diagnosis and prognosis of interstitial lung disease in autoimmune rheumatic disorders. *Ther. Adv. Musculoskel.* **2021**, *13*, 1759720X211032457. [CrossRef]
18. Krishnan, M.R.; Wang, C.M.; Marion, T.N. Anti-DNA autoantibodies initiate experimental lupus nephritis by binding directly to the glomerular basement membrane in mice. *Kidney Int.* **2012**, *82*, 184–192. [CrossRef]
19. Ahluwalia, N.; Dwyer, J.; Terry, A.; Moshfegh, A.; Johnson, C. Update on NHANES Dietary Data: Focus on Collection, Release, Analytical Considerations, and Uses to Inform Public Policy. *Adv. Nutr.* **2016**, *7*, 121–134. [CrossRef]
20. Li, Y.F.; Tang, H.; Yang, X.T.; Ma, L.L.; Zhou, H.Q.; Zhang, G.J.; Chen, X.; Ma, L.; Gao, J.; Ji, W. Associations of ω-3, ω-6 polyunsaturated fatty acids intake and ω-6: ω-3 ratio with systemic immune and inflammatory biomarkers: NHANES 1999-2020. *Front. Nutr.* **2024**, *11*, 1410154. [CrossRef]
21. Huang, S.Q.; Jiang, J.C.; Gong, H.Y. Association between dietary omega-3 fatty acid intake and all-cause mortality in patients with osteoarthritis: A population-based prospective cohort study. *Sci. Rep.* **2024**, *14*, 26516. [CrossRef] [PubMed]
22. Kang, T.; Xi, Y.; Qian, T.; Lu, S.; Du, M.; Shi, X.; Hou, X. Exploring the link between dietary omega-3 and omega-6 fatty acid intake and rheumatoid arthritis risk: NHANES 1999-2020 study. *Clin. Exp. Rheumatol.* **2024**, *42*, 1720–1728. [CrossRef] [PubMed]
23. Staruszkiewicz, M.; Pituch-Noworolska, A.; Skoczen, S. Uncommon types of autoantibodies—Detection and clinical associations. *Autoimmun. Rev.* **2023**, *22*, 103263. [CrossRef] [PubMed]

24. Somers, E.C.; Ganser, M.A.; Warren, J.S.; Basu, N.; Wang, L.; Zick, S.M.; Park, S.K. Mercury Exposure and Antinuclear Antibodies among Females of Reproductive Age in the United States: NHANES. *Environ. Health Persp.* **2015**, *123*, 792–798. [CrossRef]
25. Gui, Z.; Li, S.Y.; Yu, H.Q.; Chang, L.; Chang, Y. Sex-specific relationship between serum 25-hydroxyvitamin D concentrations and antinuclear antibodies in US adults, NHANES 2001–2004. *BMC Immunol.* **2024**, *25*, 81. [CrossRef]
26. Jiang, S.S.; Yang, W.H.; Li, Y.M.; Feng, J.Y.; Miao, J.J.; Shi, H.M.; Xue, H. Monounsaturated and polyunsaturated fatty acids concerning prediabetes and type 2 diabetes mellitus risk among participants in the National Health and Nutrition Examination Surveys (NHANES) from 2005 to March 2020. *Front. Nutr.* **2023**, *10*, 1284800. [CrossRef]
27. Che, J.H.; He, N.; Kuang, X.; Zheng, C.Y.; Zhou, R.Y.; Zhan, X.D.; Liu, Z. Dietary n-3 Fatty Acids Intake and All-Cause and Cardiovascular Mortality in Patients With Prediabetes and Diabetes. *J. Clin. Endocr. Metab.* **2024**, *109*, 2847–2856. [CrossRef]
28. Susai, S.R.; Mongan, D.; Healy, C.; Cannon, M.; Nelson, B.; Markulev, C.; Schäfer, M.R.; Berger, M.; Mossaheb, N.; Schlögelhofer, M.; et al. The association of plasma inflammatory markers with omega-3 fatty acids and their mediating role in psychotic symptoms and functioning: An analysis of the NEURAPRO clinical trial. *Brain Behav. Immun.* **2022**, *99*, 147–156. [CrossRef]
29. Abd Alhusen, S.K.; Hasan, A.F. Evaluating the renoprotective effects of omega-3-6-9 against cisplatin-induced nephrotoxicity in mice. *J. Med. Life* **2023**, *16*, 1756–1759. [CrossRef]
30. Fares, S.; Omar, M.; Laurence, A.; Abu-Baker, S.; Shaza, A.; Fadi, H.; Jonathan, M.; Georges, K.; Koushik, S.; Elie, B.S.; et al. Over-the-Counter Anti-inflammatory Supplements for Adjunctive Rheumatoid Arthritis Therapy: A Comprehensive Narrative Review. *Aging Dis.* **2025**, *16*, 408. [CrossRef]
31. Nikiphorou, E.; Philippou, E. Nutrition and its role in prevention and management of rheumatoid arthritis. *Autoimmun. Rev.* **2023**, *22*, 103333. [CrossRef] [PubMed]
32. Liu, A.L.; Li, Z.; Zeng, J.W.; Peng, Y.R.; Wang, S.; Bi, X.Y.; Zhao, Z.; Zhou, S.; Zhao, A.Z.; Mu, Y.; et al. ω-3 polyunsaturated fatty acid alleviates systemic lupus erythematosus by suppressing autoimmunity in a murine model. *Int. Immunopharmacol.* **2024**, *126*, 111299. [CrossRef] [PubMed]
33. Feng, C.L.; Li, L.Y.; Li, Q.; Switzer, K.; Liu, M.Y.; Han, S.H.; Zheng, B. Docosahexaenoic acid ameliorates autoimmune inflammation by activating GPR120 signaling pathway in dendritic cells. *Int. Immunopharmacol.* **2021**, *97*, 107698. [CrossRef] [PubMed]
34. Kim, H.K.; Kang, E.Y.; Go, G.W. Recent insights into dietary w-6 fatty acid health implications using a systematic review. *Food Sci. Biotechnol.* **2022**, *31*, 1365–1376. [CrossRef]
35. Montecillo-Aguado, M.; Tirado-Rodriguez, B.; Antonio-Andres, G.; Morales-Martinez, M.; Tong, Z.; Yang, J.; Hammock, B.D.; Hernandez-Pando, R.; Huerta-Yepez, S. Omega-6 Polyunsaturated Fatty Acids Enhance Tumor Aggressiveness in Experimental Lung Cancer Model: Important Role of Oxylipins. *Int. J. Mol. Sci.* **2022**, *23*, 6179. [CrossRef]
36. Ludovico, I.D.; Sarkar, S.; Elliott, E.; Virtanen, S.M.; Erlund, I.; Ramanadham, S.; Mirmira, R.G.; Metz, T.O.; Nakayasu, E.S. Fatty acid-mediated signaling as a target for developing type 1 diabetes therapies. *Expert Opin. Ther. Targets* **2023**, *27*, 793–806. [CrossRef]
37. Yelken, H.D.; Elci, M.P.; Turker, P.F.; Demirkaya, S. Omega fatty acid ratios and neurodegeneration in a healthy environment. *Prostaglandins Other Lipid Mediat.* **2024**, *170*, 106799. [CrossRef]
38. Wu, H.; Zhu, L.; Kinnear, D.; Triggs, N.; Quintanilla, N.M.; Himes, R. Clinical, Laboratory, and Histologic Correlates of Serum Antinuclear Antibody in Hispanic Pediatric Patients With Nonalcoholic Fatty Liver Disease. *Am. J. Clin. Pathol.* **2022**, *158*, 221–227. [CrossRef]
39. Gorczyca, D.; Szponar, B.; Pasciak, M.; Czajkowska, A.; Szmyrka, M. Serum levels of n-3 and n-6 polyunsaturated fatty acids in patients with systemic lupus erythematosus and their association with disease activity: A pilot study. *Scand. J. Rheumatol.* **2022**, *51*, 230–236. [CrossRef]
40. Endo, J.; Arita, M. Cardioprotective mechanism of omega-3 polyunsaturated fatty acids. *J. Cardiol.* **2016**, *67*, 22–27. [CrossRef]
41. Jalili, M.; Hekmatdoost, A. Dietary ω-3 fatty acids and their influence on inflammation via Toll-like receptor pathways. *Nutrition* **2021**, *85*, 111070. [CrossRef] [PubMed]
42. Hellwing, C.; Schoeniger, A.; Roessler, C.; Leimert, A.; Schumann, J. Lipid raft localization of TLR2 and its co-receptors is independent of membrane lipid composition. *PeerJ* **2018**, *6*, e4212. [CrossRef] [PubMed]
43. Schoeniger, A.; Fuhrmann, H.; Schumann, J. LPS- or *Pseudomonas aeruginosa*-mediated activation of the macrophage TLR4 signaling cascade depends on membrane lipid composition. *PeerJ* **2016**, *4*, e1663. [CrossRef] [PubMed]
44. Xia, Y.; Zhang, Y.; Li, Y.; Li, X.; Wu, Y.; Yao, Q. Omega-3 polyunsaturated fatty acids play a protective role in a mouse model of Parkinson's disease by increasing intestinal inducible Treg cells. *Cell. Mol. Biol.* **2024**, *70*, 107–112. [CrossRef]
45. Pauls, S.D.; Rodway, L.A.; Winter, T.; Taylor, C.G.; Zahradka, P.; Aukema, H.M. Anti-inflammatory effects of α-linolenic acid in M1-like macrophages are associated with enhanced production of oxylipins from α-linolenic and linoleic acid. *J. Nutr. Biochem.* **2018**, *57*, 121–129. [CrossRef]
46. Montserrat-de La Paz, S.; Naranjo, M.C.; Lopez, S.; Abia, R.; Muriana, F.; Bermudez, B. Niacin and olive oil promote skewing to the M2 phenotype in bone marrow-derived macrophages of mice with metabolic syndrome. *Food Funct.* **2016**, *7*, 2233–2238. [CrossRef]

47. Chung, M.Y.; Kim, B.H. Fatty acids and epigenetics in health and diseases. *Food Sci. Biotechnol.* **2024**, *33*, 3153–3166. [CrossRef]
48. Aslibekyan, S.; Wiener, H.W.; Have, P.J.; Stanhope, K.L.; O'Brien, D.M.; Hopkins, S.E.; Absher, D.M.; Tiwari, H.K.; Boyer, B.B. DNA Methylation Patterns Are Associated with n-3 Fatty Acid Intake in Yup'ik People. *J. Nutr.* **2014**, *144*, 425–430. [CrossRef]
49. Ahlberg, E.; Martí, M.; Govindaraj, D.; Severin, E.; Duchén, K.; Jenmalm, M.C.; Tingö, L. Immune-related microRNAs in breast milk and their relation to regulatory T cells in breastfed children. *Pediatr. Allergy Immunol.* **2023**, *34*, e13952. [CrossRef]
50. Abrescia, P.; Treppiccione, L.; Rossi, M.; Bergamo, P. Modulatory role of dietary polyunsaturated fatty acids in Nrf2-mediated redox homeostasis. *Prog. Lipid Res.* **2020**, *80*, 101066. [CrossRef]
51. Zhu, X.L.; Bi, Z.C.; Yang, C.; Guo, Y.H.; Yuan, J.L.; Li, L.J.; Guo, Y. Effects of different doses of omega-3 polyunsaturated fatty acids on gut microbiota and immunity. *Food Nutr. Res.* **2021**, *65*, 6263. [CrossRef]
52. Fu, Y.W.; Wang, Y.D.; Gao, H.; Li, D.H.; Jiang, R.R.; Ge, L.R.; Tong, C.; Xu, K. Associations among Dietary Omega-3 Polyunsaturated Fatty Acids, the Gut Microbiota, and Intestinal Immunity. *Mediat. Inflamm.* **2021**, *2021*, 8879227. [CrossRef]

nutrients

MDPI

Article

The Inhibitory Effects of NCT503 and Exogenous Serine on High-Selenium Induced Insulin Resistance in Mice

Shuo Zhan [1], Jianrong Wang [1], Mingyu Zhu [1], Yiqun Liu [1], Feng Han [1], Licui Sun [1], Qin Wang [1,*] and Zhenwu Huang [1,2,*]

1 National Institute for Nutrition and Health, Chinese Center for Disease Control and Prevention, Beijing 100050, China; zs_peipei@outlook.com (S.Z.); jianrongwang666@163.com (J.W.); z18846757274@163.com (M.Z.); liuyq@ninh.chinacdc.cn (Y.L.); hanfeng@ninh.chinacdc.cn (F.H.); sunlc@ninh.chinacdc.cn (L.S.)

2 Key Laboratory of Public Nutrition and Health, National Health Commission of the People's Republic of China, Beijing 100050, China

* Correspondence: wangqin@ninh.chinacdc.cn (Q.W.); huangzw@ninh.chinacdc.cn (Z.H.)

Abstract: Objective: This study aims to identify whether the development of insulin resistance (IR) induced by high selenium (Se) is related to serine deficiency via the inhibition of the de novo serine synthesis pathway (SSP) by the administrations of 3-phosphoglycerate dehydrogenase (PHGDH) inhibitor (NCT503) or exogenous serine in mice. Method: forty-eight male C57BL/6J mice were randomly divided into four groups: adequate-Se (0.1 mgSe/kg), high-Se (0.8 mgSe/kg), high-Se +serine (240 mg/kg/day), and high-Se +NCT503 (30 mg/kg, twice a week) for 5 months. The glucose tolerance test (GTT) and insulin tolerance test (ITT) were used to confirm the development of IR in mice with high-Se intake, and fasting blood glucose levels were measured monthly. The Se contents in plasma and tissues were detected by ICP-MS. The levels of insulin (INS), homocysteine (HCY), and serine in plasma were tested by ELISA. Western blot analyses were conducted to evaluate the protein expressions of glutathione peroxidase 1 (GPX1), selenoprotein P (SELENOP) and PHGDH, the PI3K-AKT-mTOR pathway, folate cycle (SHMT1, MTHFR), and methionine cycle (MS). Results: An IR model was developed in mice from the high-Se group with elevated fasting blood glucose and INS levels, impaired glucose tolerance, and reduced insulin sensitivity, but not in both the high-Se +serine group and the high-Se +NCT503 group. Compared with the high-Se and high-Se +serine groups, the expressions of GPX1 and SELENOP significantly decreased for the high-Se +NCT503 group in the liver, muscle, and pancreas tissues. The expression of PHGDH of high-Se group was significantly higher than that of the adequate-Se group in the liver ($p < 0.05$) and pancreas ($p < 0.001$). Also, the expected high expression of PHGDH was effectively inhibited in mice from the high-Se +serine group but not from the high-Se +NCT503 group. The expression of p-AKT (Ser-473) for the high-Se group was significantly lower than that of the adequate-Se group in the liver, muscle, and pancreas. Conclusions: The IR induced by high-Se intake in the body has been confirmed to be partially due to serine deficiency, which led to the initiation of SSP to produce endogenous serine. The supplementations of exogenous serine or inhibitors of PHGDH in this metabolic pathway could be used for the intervention.

Keywords: high-Se; IR; SSP; PHGDH inhibitor; serine

1. Introduction

Selenium is an essential trace mineral with critical roles in maintaining physiological homeostasis. As a vital component of selenoproteins, such as glutathione peroxidases

(GPX) and thioredoxin reductases, selenium protects cells against oxidative stress and contributes to redox balance [1]. It also plays a key role in thyroid hormone metabolism, where Se-dependent enzymes regulate the activation and breakdown of thyroid hormones, and in modulating immune responses and inflammatory processes.

Dietary selenium is derived from various natural sources, including Brazil nuts, seafood, organ meats, poultry, eggs, and cereals. However, the selenium content of foods varies significantly by geographic region due to differences in soil selenium levels. The recommended dietary allowance (RDA) for selenium is 55 μg/day for adults, with increased requirements for pregnant (60 μg/day) and lactating women (70 μg/day). The tolerable upper intake level (UL) is 400 μg/day, beyond which adverse effects may occur.

While selenium deficiency is rare in most healthy populations, certain groups—such as individuals consuming Se-poor diets, patients with gastrointestinal disorders, or those dependent on parenteral nutrition—are at increased risk. Selenium deficiency can lead to diseases, such as Keshan disease (cardiomyopathy) and Kashin-Beck disease (osteoarthropathy), as well as impaired immune function and thyroid dysfunction.

Conversely, excessive selenium intake poses significant health risks. Chronic or acute selenium toxicity (selenosis) can result from consumption exceeding the UL, particularly through over-supplementation or dietary excess. Symptoms of selenosis include garlic breath odor, brittle hair and nails, gastrointestinal distress, fatigue, irritability, and neurological damage. In severe cases, selenium toxicity can lead to organ failure or death.

Beyond its toxic effects, supranutritional selenium intake has been increasingly linked to metabolic disorders, including insulin resistance (IR) and type 2 diabetes (T2D). IR is an important factor in the progression of T2D [2]. Large-scale studies in North America have associated excessive selenium intake with increased diabetes risk, potentially due to oxidative stress and disruption of insulin signaling pathways. These findings highlight selenium's dual role in health, where adequate levels are essential for metabolic and cellular functions, but excessive levels drive metabolic dysregulation.

As early as 2004, hallmark features of T2D, including pancreatic hypertrophy, hyperinsulinemia, hyperglycemia, and obesity were developed in GPX1-overexpressing transgenic mice fed with 0.4 mgSe/kg diet [3]. Interestingly, when these mice were switched to a low-Se diet (<0.02 mgSe/kg) [4], most symptoms, except for hyperinsulinemia, were partially alleviated or disappeared.

In 2010, another research team from Japan found that selenoprotein P (SELENOP), synthesized by the liver and secreted into the bloodstream, also interfered with the normal signaling of insulin and disrupted glucose metabolism in cultured hepatic cells and skeletal muscle cells [5]. In vivo, the same research team first injected purified human SELENOP directly into mice and observed the occurrence of IR, which was relieved by administering a neutralizing antibody against human SELENOP [6].

Meanwhile, IR models have been successfully developed in different animals by feeding with high-Se diets naturally [7]. For example, Vyacheslav et al. reported that feeding male C57BL/6J mice a 0.4 mg/kg Se diet led to hyperinsulinemia and reduced insulin sensitivity, accompanied by a slight increase in the expression of certain selenoproteins [8]. Similarly, Zeng et al. observed IR-like features in pregnant Wistar rats and their offspring when fed a 3 mg/kg Se diet, with a concurrent increase in GPX1 expression [9].

The mechanistic basis for Se-induced abnormal glucose metabolism was first proposed by Lei Xingen's research group [10,11], who identified IR as a key feature. This was attributed to the disruption of insulin signaling pathways due to low hydrogen peroxide (H_2O_2) levels, a consequence of the overexpression of antioxidant selenoproteins, such as GPX1 [12].

We previously reported that serine enhances selenoprotein expression in cultured cells [13], and discovered that disruptions in endogenous serine synthesis significantly impact selenoprotein expression in maternal tissues and subsequent offspring development [14]. These findings were further validated in vivo using a high-Se-induced IR mouse model [15], suggesting a potential link to the SESAME complex, which comprises S-adenosylmethionine (SAM) and various enzymes involved in glycolysis, serine synthesis, folate cycle, and methionine cycle [16].

Excessive selenium in the body leads to the accumulation of hydrogen selenide (H_2Se), which must be methylated by SAM to be efficiently excreted as CH_3^-SeSUG or $(CH_3)_3Se^+$. Without adequate SAM, severe toxic effects can occur. It has been observed that selenium toxicity in animals depletes SAM, which in turn leads to the depletion of serine, as recent studies suggest that synthesizing a single SAM molecule may consume a great amount of serine [17,18].

This study aimed to observe the inhibition effect of exogenous serine or a PHGDH inhibitor (NCT-503) on the activation of the serine synthesis pathway (SSP) in mice fed with high-Se, which provided a possible intervention for T2D induced by high-Se.

2. Materials and Methods

2.1. Reagents

Glucose, insulin, serine, primary antibodies (β-actin, PI3K, GPX1, SELENOP, SELENON, SHMT1, and MS), and HRP-conjugated IgG were sourced from Sigma-Aldrich (Shanghai, China). P-Akt (Ser473, Thr308), PHGDH, and MTHFR antibodies came from Abcam (Shanghai, China); mTOR and Akt antibodies were from Cell Signaling Technology (Denver, CO, USA). Additional chemicals were obtained from Wako Pure Chemical and Hitachi Co. (Osaka, Japan). The PHGDH inhibitor NCT-503 was provided by Shanghai Haoyuan (Shanghai, China) (MedChem Express). The ECL solution, Blue Plus II Protein Marker, and EasySee Western Marker were acquired from TransGen Biotech (Beijing, China).

2.2. Experimental Groups and Diet Regimes

Figure 1 presents an outline of the animal experimental design. Forty-eight male C57BL/6J mice, aged 4 weeks and maintained at SPF status, were obtained from Beijing SBF Biotech Co., Ltd., Beijing, China, and housed under standard conditions. The temperature was maintained at 24 °C, and the relative humidity was kept at 55%. Following a one-week acclimation, mice were randomly assigned to four groups (n = 12): adequate-Se (0.1 mg Se/kg), high-Se (0.8 mg Se/kg), high-Se +serine (240 mg/kg/day), and high-Se +NCT503 (30 mg/kg, twice a week). The serine intervention group was fed with continuous 0.8 mg/kg Se and given serine by intragastric administration (240 mg/kg/day) [14,19]. NCT-503 was prepared by sequentially adding 10% DMSO (Sigma), 40% PEG300 (Sigma), 5% Tween-80 (Sigma), and 45% saline and administered intraperitoneally at a dose of 30 mg/kg twice weekly [20], with the injection volume kept below 150 μL per mouse.

The animal fodder was sourced under license SCXK (Beijing) 2024-0001. The composition of the food is provided in Table 1. The actual selenium contents measured by ICP-MS were 0.113 mg/kg for the adequate-Se group and 0.834 mg/kg for the high-Se groups. According to reference [7], glucose tolerance tests (GTTs) and insulin tolerance tests (ITTs) were conducted on mice starting from the fourth month. One month after IR was observed in the high-Se group, blood was collected from the retro-orbital sinus, mice were sacrificed, and target tissues were collected within 5 min to preserve their metabolic state. Tissue samples were stored at −80 °C.

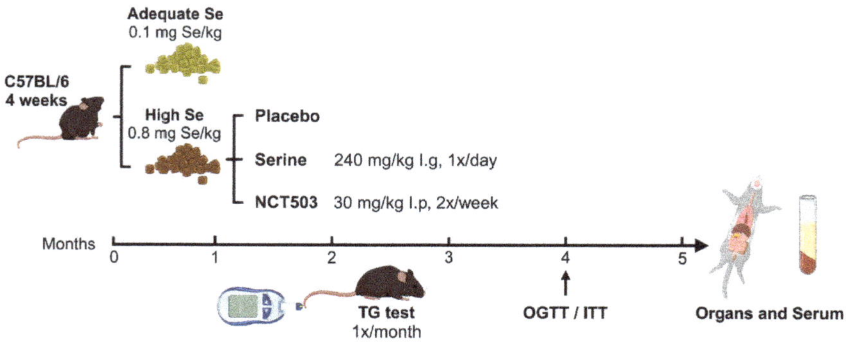

Figure 1. Animal experiment flowchart.

Table 1. Diet composition with selenium content (unit/kg) for mice.

	Adequate-Se (0.1 mg/kg)	High-Se (0.8 mg/kg)
L-alanine	0.35	0.35
L-arginine	1.21	1.21
L-asparagine	0.6	0.6
L-aspartic acid	0.35	0.35
L-cysteine	0.35	0.35
L-glutamic acid	4	4
Glycine	2.33	2.33
L-his	0.45	0.45
L-isoleucine	0.82	0.82
L-methionine	0.82	0.82
L-leucine	1.11	1.11
L-Lysine hydrochloride	1.8	1.8
L-Phenylalanine	0.75	0.75
L-proline	0.35	0.35
L-serine	0.35	0.35
L-threonine	0.82	0.82
L-Tryptophan	0.18	0.18
L-Tyrosine	0.5	0.5
L-valine	0.82	0.82
Corn starch	15	15
Maltodextrin	15	15
Sucrose	35.17	35.17
Cellulose	3	3
Soybean oil	8	8
Choline Bitartrate	0.25	0.25
Calcium hydrogen phosphate	0.82	0.82
AIN mineral mixture	3.5	3.5
AIN Vitamin Mix	1.3	1.3
Sodium selenite	0.02190 g	0.175267 g
Total	100	100

2.3. Weekly Body Weight Monitoring in C57BL/6J Mice

Weekly body weight measurements were taken for C57BL/6J mice throughout the 5-month study period. Mice were weighed at the same time each week using a digital scale. The mice were fed diets containing 0.1 or 0.8 mg Se/kg, and body weight changes were recorded to assess the effects of different treatments.

2.4. Glucose Tolerance Test (GTT)

Measure blood glucose levels in the tail vein of mice using a blood glucose meter (Johnson & Johnson, Shanghai, China). Mice underwent a 12 h fast before receiving a glucose injection (1 mg/g) for the GTT, with an injection volume not exceeding 200 µL. Blood glucose levels were recorded at 0, 20, 30, 60, and 120 min.

2.5. Insulin Tolerance Test (ITT)

In the ITTs, mice were fasted for 12 h. Insulin (0.75 mU/g body weight) [21] was then administered intraperitoneally, with an injection volume not exceeding 200 µL. Tail vein blood glucose levels were measured at 0, 30, 60, 120, and 240 min.

2.6. Fasting Blood Glucose Test

Fasting blood glucose in the mice was monitored monthly. Following a 12 h overnight fast, tail vein blood samples were directly measured using a glucometer (Johnson & Johnson, Shanghai, China). Data were recorded as blood glucose concentrations at the time of measurement.

2.7. Selenium Detection of Plasma and Tissues in Mice

Plasma and tissue selenium levels were determined using microwave digestion with nitric acid, followed by analysis via inductively coupled plasma mass spectrometry (ICP-MS), as previously described [22].

2.8. Blood Biochemistry Analysis

Plasma levels of insulin (INS), homocysteine (HCY), and serine were measured using commercial ELISA kits, employing a double-antibody sandwich method for enzyme-linked immunosor. All assays were conducted following the manufacturer's protocols.

2.9. PHGDH Enzyme Activity Assay

The enzyme activity of PHGDH was determined using an ELISA kit (Jiangsu Jingmei Biological technology Co., Ltd., Yancheng, China), following the manufacturer's instructions. Samples were processed and analyzed as per the provided protocol. Absorbance (OD values) were measured at a wavelength of 450 nm using a microplate reader, and enzyme activity was calculated accordingly.

2.10. Western Blotting

Protein extraction, SDS-PAGE, membrane transfer, antibody incubation, and ECL detection were performed following standard protocols [23].

2.11. Statistical Analysis

Data are presented as mean ± Standard Deviation (SD). Graphs were generated using GraphPad Prism 9.0, and statistical analyses were performed with SPSS 20.0 software (SPSS Inc., Chicago, IL, USA). Group comparisons were evaluated using analysis of variance (ANOVA), followed by post hoc comparisons using the Sidak test. Prior to applying ANOVA, the assumptions of normality and homogeneity of variances were assessed using the Shapiro–Wilk test and Levene's test, respectively. If the data violated the assumption of normality, the non-parametric Kruskal–Wallis test was employed. If heteroscedasticity was detected, Welch's ANOVA was used instead of the standard ANOVA.

3. Results

3.1. Weekly Body Weight Monitoring

C57BL/6J mice were intervened, as shown in Figure 1 and Table S1, for 5 months, with body weight monitored weekly. Supplementation with Ser or NCT503 significantly reduced the Se-induced weight gain (**** $p < 0.0001$ and * $p < 0.05$, respectively), with the NCT503 group's weight closer to that of the control group. The Ser group exhibited a markedly greater reduction in body weight than the NCT503 group (**** $p < 0.0001$) (Figure 2a).

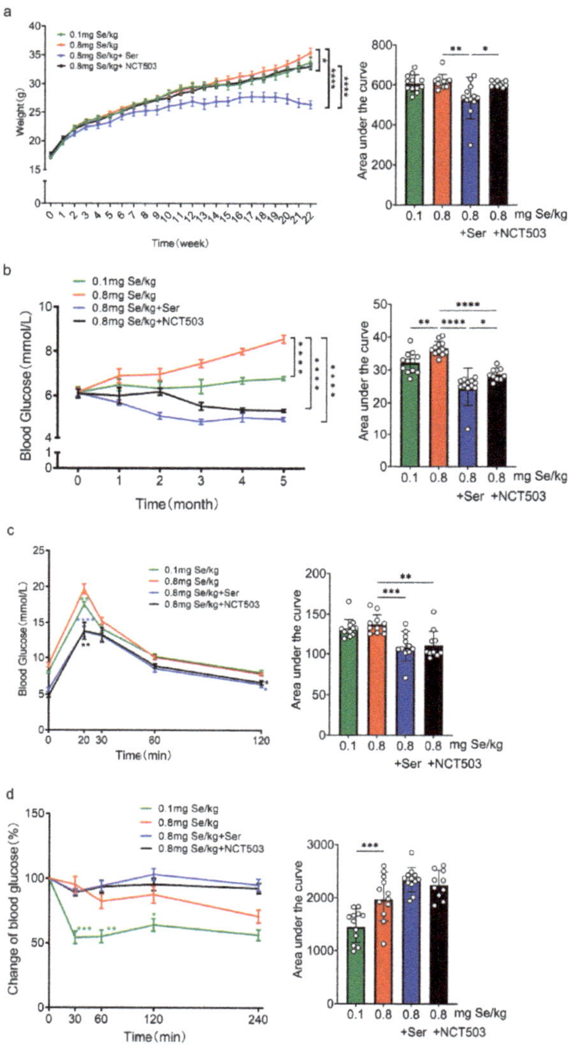

Figure 2. Effects of selenium levels (0.1, 0.8 mg Se/kg) and interventions (Ser, NCT503) on weight, glucose metabolism, GTT, and ITT in C57BL/6J mice. (**a**) Changes in body weight over 5 months. (**b**) Fasting blood glucose levels measured monthly. (**c**) Glucose tolerance assessed at the end of the fourth month. (**d**) Insulin tolerance evaluated at the end of the fourth month. (Data are expressed as mean ± SD, n = 10–12). (* $p < 0.05$, ** $p < 0.01$, *** $p < 0.001$, **** $p < 0.0001$; two-way ANOVA). Both Ser and NCT503 effectively mitigate Se-induced metabolic disturbances, with Ser showing a more substantial improvement in body weight and blood glucose regulation.

3.2. Monthly Monitoring of Fasting Blood Glucose Levels

Mice were fed, as shown in Figure 2 and Table S1, for 5 months. Fasting blood glucose levels (tail vein blood after a 12 h fast) were monitored monthly. Mice of the 0.8 mg Se/kg group exhibited a gradual increase in blood glucose levels, reaching a peak at the fifth month (**** $p < 0.0001$) compared to the adequate-Se group. Supplementation with Ser or NCT503 improved fasting glucose levels gradually, which reached the lowest point at the fifth month compared to the high-Se group alone (**** $p < 0.0001$) (Figure 2b).

3.3. Glucose Tolerance Test

After a 4-month intervention, blood glucose levels were evaluated at specified time points following glucose injection (1 mg/g). Mice of the 0.8 mg Se/kg group exhibited significantly elevated blood glucose levels at 20 min compared to the 0.1 mg Se/kg group (** $p < 0.01$). Supplementation with Ser or NCT503 significantly improved glucose tolerance, resulting in lower blood glucose levels compared to the 0.8 mg Se/kg group alone (**** $p < 0.0001$ and ** $p < 0.01$, respectively) (Figure 2c and Table S1).

3.4. Insulin Tolerance Test

Mice were administered for 4 months. ITTs were performed, and the data were expressed as percentage changes from baseline. As illustrated in Figure 2d and Table S1, 30 min after insulin injection, the percentage change in blood glucose was significantly higher in the 0.8 mg Se/kg group compared to the 0.1 mg Se/kg group (*** $p < 0.001$). The elevated glucose response persisted at 60 and 120 min (** $p < 0.01$ and * $p < 0.05$, respectively), with no significant differences observed between the Ser and NCT503 groups.

3.5. High Se and Ser/NCT503 Supplementation Differentially Modulate Plasma Biochemical Markers

As shown in Figure 3a and Table S2, INS levels were significantly elevated in the 0.8 mg Se/kg group compared to the 0.1 mg Se/kg group (**** $p < 0.0001$). Supplementary with Ser or NCT503 resulted in a significant reduction in INS levels (**** $p < 0.0001$). Figure 3b and Table S2 show that HCY levels were significantly lower in the 0.8 mg Se/kg group compared to the 0.1 mg Se/kg group (*** $p < 0.001$). Supplementation with serine further reduced HCY levels (**** $p < 0.0001$), whereas NCT503 intervention significantly increased HCY levels (**** $p < 0.0001$). In Figure 3c and Table S2, serine levels were significantly higher in the 0.8 mg Se/kg group compared to the 0.1 mg Se/kg group (*** $p < 0.001$). NCT503 supplementation significantly decreased serine levels (**** $p < 0.0001$) compared to the 0.8 mg Se/kg group, while serine supplementation slightly increased serine levels, although the change was not statistically significant.

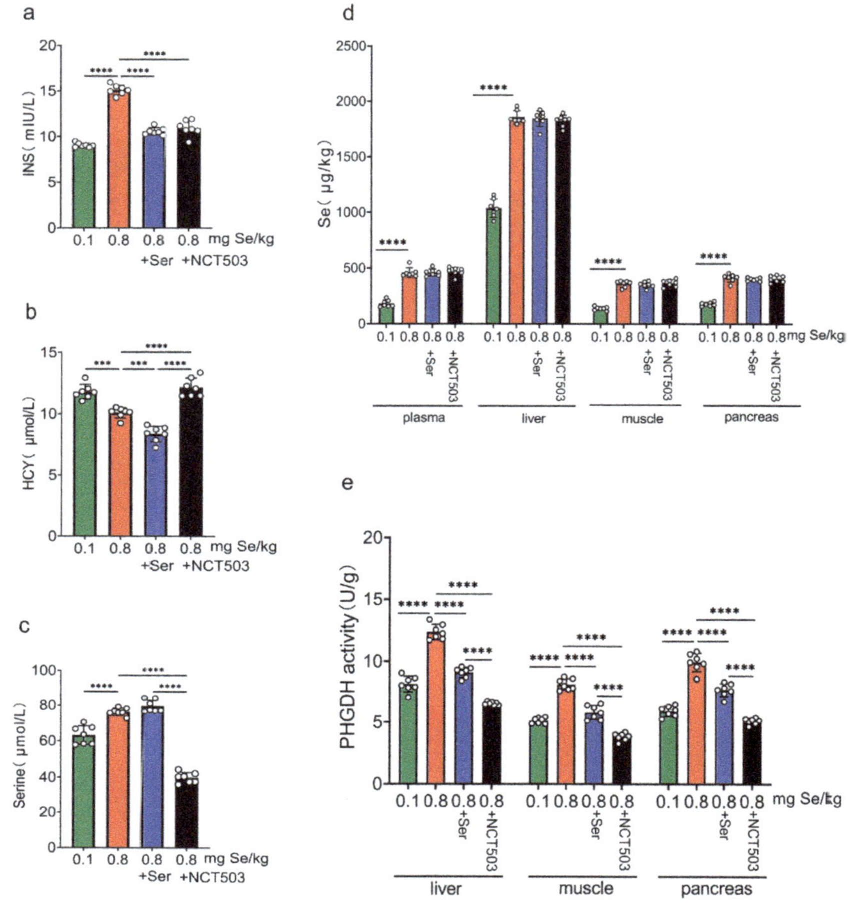

Figure 3. Effects of selenium levels (0.1 mg and 0.8 mg Se/kg) and interventions (Ser, NCT503) on plasma biochemical markers in C57BL/6J mice. (**a–c**) Changes in plasma biochemical markers: (**a**) insulin (INS, mIU/L), (**b**) homocysteine (Hcy, μmol/L), amd (**c**) serine (Ser, μmol/L). (**d**) Selenium levels in plasma, liver, muscle, and pancreas. (**e**) PHGDH enzyme activity in plasma, liver, muscle, and pancreas. (Data are expressed as mean ± SD, n = 7). (*** $p < 0.001$, **** $p < 0.0001$; two-way ANOVA). Supplementation with Ser and NCT503 modulates biochemical markers and PHGDH enzyme activity. Ser supplementation lowers INS and HCY levels, while NCT503 decreases INS and serine levels, and increases HCY levels. The NCT503 inhibitor has a stronger inhibitory effect on PHGDH enzyme activity.

3.6. Selenium Levels in Plasma, Liver, Muscle, and Pancreas

In the 0.8 mg Se/kg group, selenium concentrations in plasma, liver, muscle, and pancreas were markedly higher than those in the 0.1 mg Se/kg group (**** $p < 0.0001$). Selenium concentrations showed no significant variation with Ser or NCT503 supplementation (Figure 3d and Table S3).

3.7. PHGDH Activities in Liver, Muscle, and Pancreas

In the 0.8 mg Se/kg group, PHGDH enzyme activity in the liver, muscle, and pancreas was significantly higher than in the 0.1 mg Se/kg group (**** $p < 0.0001$). After supplementation with Ser or NCT503, PHGDH activity was markedly reduced (**** $p < 0.0001$). However, in the Ser intervention group, PHGDH activity was significantly higher than in the 0.1 mg Se/kg group (muscle: * $p < 0.05$; liver: ** $p < 0.01$; pancreas: ***** $p < 0.0001$). In contrast, PHGDH activity in the NCT503 intervention group was significantly lower than in the 0.1 mg Se/kg group (liver and muscle: **** $p < 0.0001$; pancreas: * $p < 0.05$). Furthermore, when comparing the Ser intervention group to the NCT503 group, PHGDH activity in the NCT503 group was also significantly reduced (**** $p < 0.0001$) (Figure 3e and Table S4).

3.8. Influence of Dietary Selenium Supplementation on the Expressions of Selenoproteins and Enzymes Related with Serine Metabolism in Mice Tissues

Liver. As shown in Figure 4 and Table S5, compared with the 0.1 mg Se/kg group, the expressions of GPX1, SELENOP, PHGDH, SHMT1, MTHFR, and MS were significantly higher for the 0.8 mg Se/kg group (MS, *** $p < 0.001$; SHMT1 and MTHFR, ** $p < 0.01$; GPX1, SELENOP and PHGDH, * $p < 0.05$). Mice in the Ser group showed a significant reduction in MS expression compared to the 0.8 mgSe group alone (MS, ** $p < 0.01$), while GPX1 and SELENOP expressions increased slightly, PHGDH, SHMT1, and MTHFR expressions decreased slightly, but these changes were not statistically significant. SELENOP expression (* $p < 0.05$) showed significant reductions in the NCT503 group compared to the 0.8 mgSe group. Compared to the Ser group, the expressions of GPX1 and SELENOP were lower (* $p < 0.05$), while the expressions of PHGDH were increased (* $p < 0.05$) in the NCT503 group.

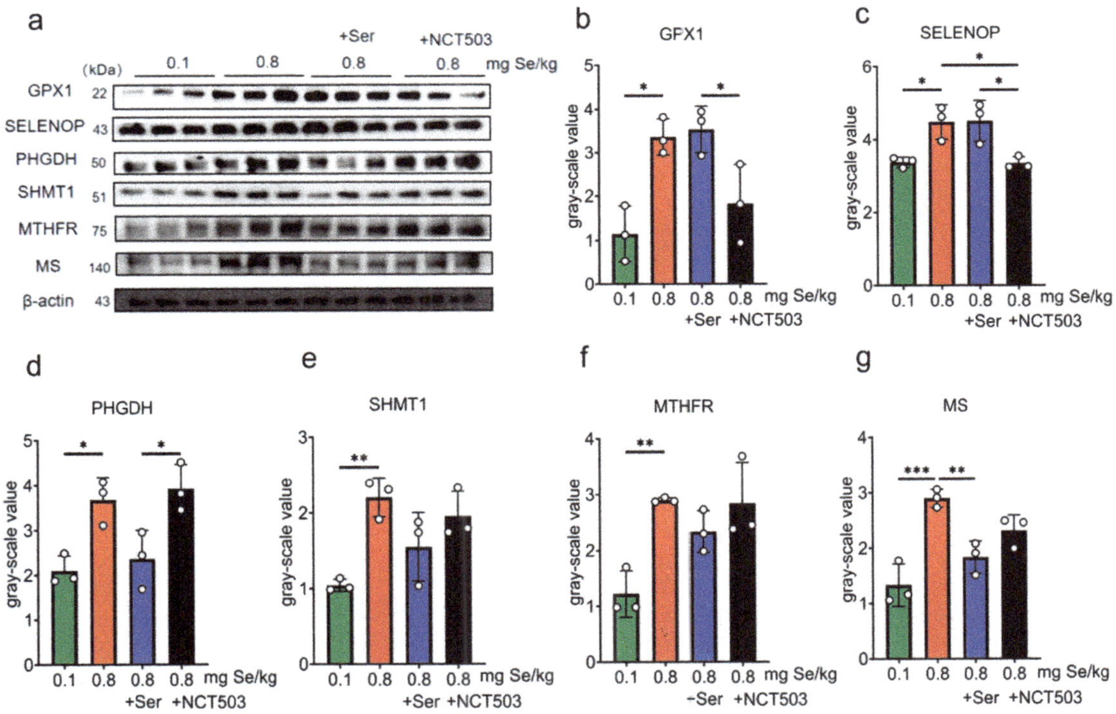

Figure 4. Effect of 0.1, 0.8 mg Se/kg and Ser or NCT503 intervention group on the Expressions of selenoproteins and enzymes in Liver Tissue. (**a**) WB images. (**b**–**g**) grayscale analysis. (Mean ± SD, n = 3, * $p < 0.05$, ** $p < 0.01$, *** $p < 0.001$; two-way ANOVA). NCT503 and Ser differentially modulate liver enzyme expression, with NCT503 enhancing PHGDH activity and reducing SELENOP, while Ser primarily decreases MS expression.

Muscle. As shown in Figure 5 and Table S6, compared with the 0.8 mgSe group, the expressions of GPX1, SELENON, MTHFR, and MS were significantly higher for the 0.1 mgSe group (GPX1, *** $p < 0.001$; SELENON, MS, ** $p < 0.01$; MTHFR, * $p < 0.05$), while the expressions of PHGDH, SHMT1 increased slightly with no statistical significance. The expressions of MS in the Ser group showed significant reductions (MS, *** $p < 0.001$) compared with 0.8 mgSe alone. For the 0.8 mgSe group, the expressions of GPX1, SELENON, and MS decreased significantly compared to NCT503 group (MS, ** $p < 0.01$; GPX1 and SELENOP, * $p < 0.05$). Protein expressions were lower in the NCT503 group compared to the Ser group (SELENOP, ** $p < 0.01$; and GPX1, * $p < 0.05$).

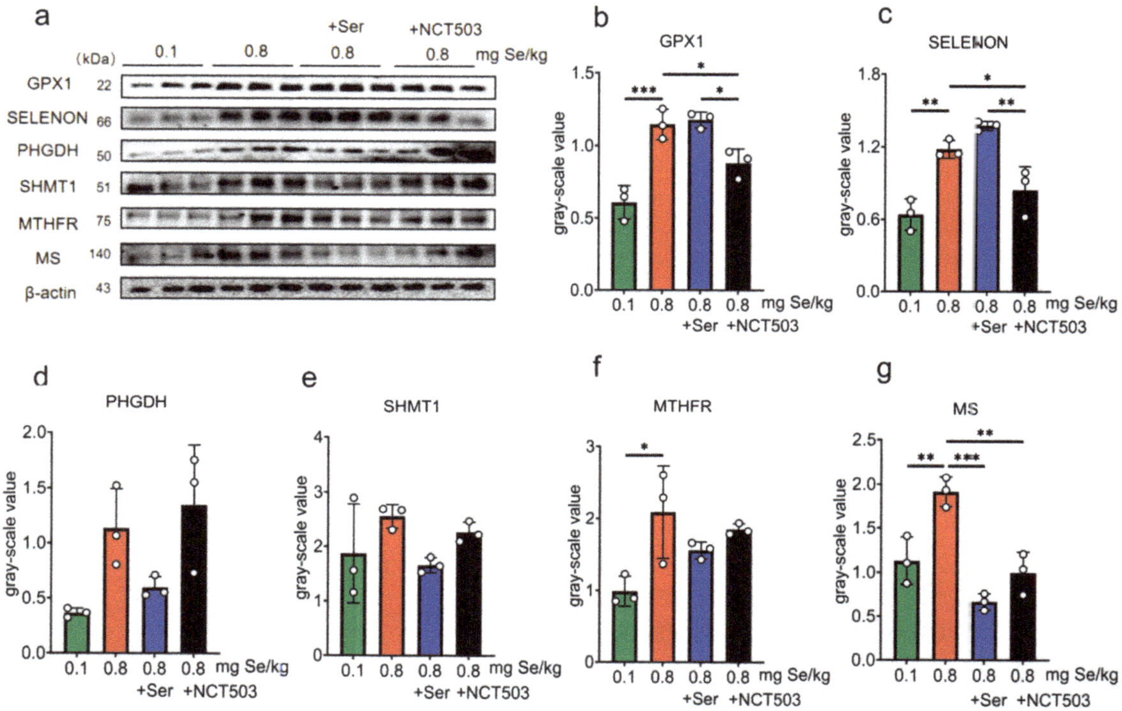

Figure 5. Effect of 0.1, 0.8 mg Se/kg and Ser or the NCT503 intervention group on the expressions of selenoproteins and enzymes in muscle Tissue. (**a**) WB images. (**b–g**) grayscale analysis. (Mean ± SD, n = 3, * $p < 0.05$, ** $p < 0.01$, *** $p < 0.001$; two-way ANOVA). NCT503 reduces GPX1 and SELENOP expression in muscle, while Ser mainly reduces MS expression.

Pancreas. As shown in Figure 6 and Table S7, for the 0.8 mgSe group, the expressions of PHGDH, SHMT1, and MS were significantly elevated compared to the 0.1 mgSe group (PHGDH, *** $p < 0.001$; MS, ** $p < 0.01$; SHMT1, * $p < 0.05$). The expression of SHMT1 showed significant reductions for the Ser group compared to the 0.8 mgSe group alone (SHMT1, * $p < 0.05$), while the expressions of GPX1 increased slightly, and PHGDH, MTHFR, and MS decreased slightly with no statistical significance. Compared to the Ser group, the expressions of GPX1 (*** $p < 0.001$) decreased, and PHGDH, SHMT1 increased (PHGDH and SHMT1,** $p < 0.01$) for the NCT503 group.

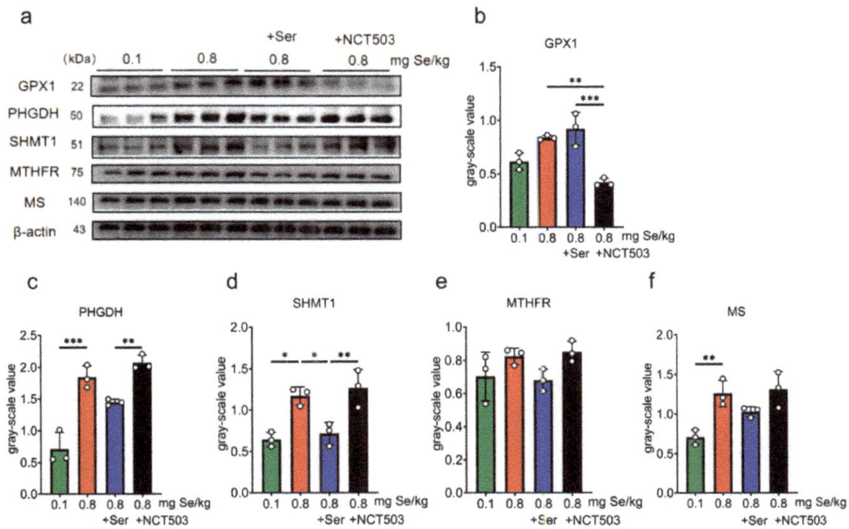

Figure 6. Effect of 0.1, 0.8 mg Se/kg and Ser or the NCT503 intervention group on the expression of selenoproteins and enzymes in Mouse pancreas Tissue. (**a**) WB images. (**b–f**) grayscale analysis. (Mean ± SD, n = 3, * $p < 0.05$, ** $p < 0.01$, *** $p < 0.001$; two-way ANOVA). NCT503 increases PHGDH expression in the pancreas, while Ser primarily reduces SHMT1 expression.

3.9. Influence of Dietary Selenium Supplementation on the PI3K-AKT-mTOR Insulin Signaling Pathway in Mouse Tissues

Liver. As shown in Figure 7 and Table S5, the expression of phosphorylated Akt1 at Ser-473 (P-Akt (Ser-473)) was significantly lower in the 0.8 mg Se/kg group than in the 0.1 mg Se/kg group (*** $p < 0.001$); the expressions of mTOR, AKT, phosphorylated Akt1 at Thr-308 (P-Akt (Thr-308)), and PI3K were slightly decreased, but these changes were not statistically significant. Compared to the 0.8 mg Se/kg group, the expressions of mTOR increased significantly in the 0.8 mgSe/kg +Ser and 0.8 mg Se/kg +NCT503 groups (* $p < 0.05$). The expressions of AKT, P-Akt (Ser-473), P-Akt (Thr-308), and PI3K showed slight increases, but these were not statistically significant.

Muscle. As shown in Figure 8 and Table S6, mTOR, P-Akt (Ser-473), and PI3K expression levels were significantly lower in the 0.8 mg Se/kg group compared to the 0.1 mg Se/kg group (* $p < 0.05$). The expressions of AKT and P-Akt (Thr-308) were slightly decreased, but these changes were not statistically significant. Compared to the 0.8 mg Se/kg group, the expressions of mTOR, AKT, P-Akt (Ser-473), P-Akt (Thr-308), and PI3K in the 0.8 mg Se/kg +Ser or 0.8 mg Se/kg +NCT503 group showed slight increases, but these were not statistically significant.

Pancreas. As shown in Figure 9 and Table S7, the 0.8 mg Se/kg group exhibited significantly reduced expressions of mTOR, P-Akt (Ser-473), and P-Akt (Thr-308) compared to the 0.1 mg Se/kg group (*** $p < 0.001$). The expressions of AKT and PI3K were slightly lower, but these changes were not statistically significant. The expressions of mTOR and P-Akt (Ser-473) increased significantly in the 0.8 mg Se/kg +Ser group (*** $p < 0.001$) compared to the 0.8 mg Se/kg group, while the expressions of AKT, P-Akt (Thr-308), and PI3K showed slight, non-significant increases. Similarly, compared to the 0.8 mg Se/kg group, the expressions of mTOR, P-Akt (Ser-473) (*** $p < 0.001$), and P-Akt (Thr-308) (** $p < 0.01$) were significantly increased in the 0.8 mg Se/kg +NCT503 group, while the expressions of AKT and PI3K showed slight, non-significant increases.

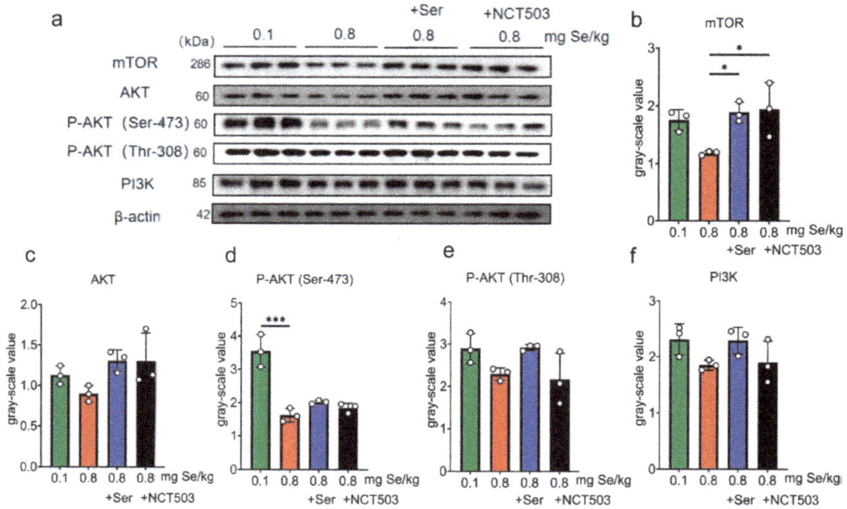

Figure 7. Effects of 0.1, 0.8 mg Se/kg, and Ser or the NCT503 intervention group on the PI3K-AKT-mTOR pathway in mice liver. (**a**) WB images. (**b–f**) Pathway grayscale analysis (Mean ± SD, n = 3, * $p < 0.05$, *** $p < 0.001$; two-way ANOVA). Ser and NCT503 supplementation modulate mTOR expression in the liver, with NCT503 and Ser both enhancing mTOR signaling.

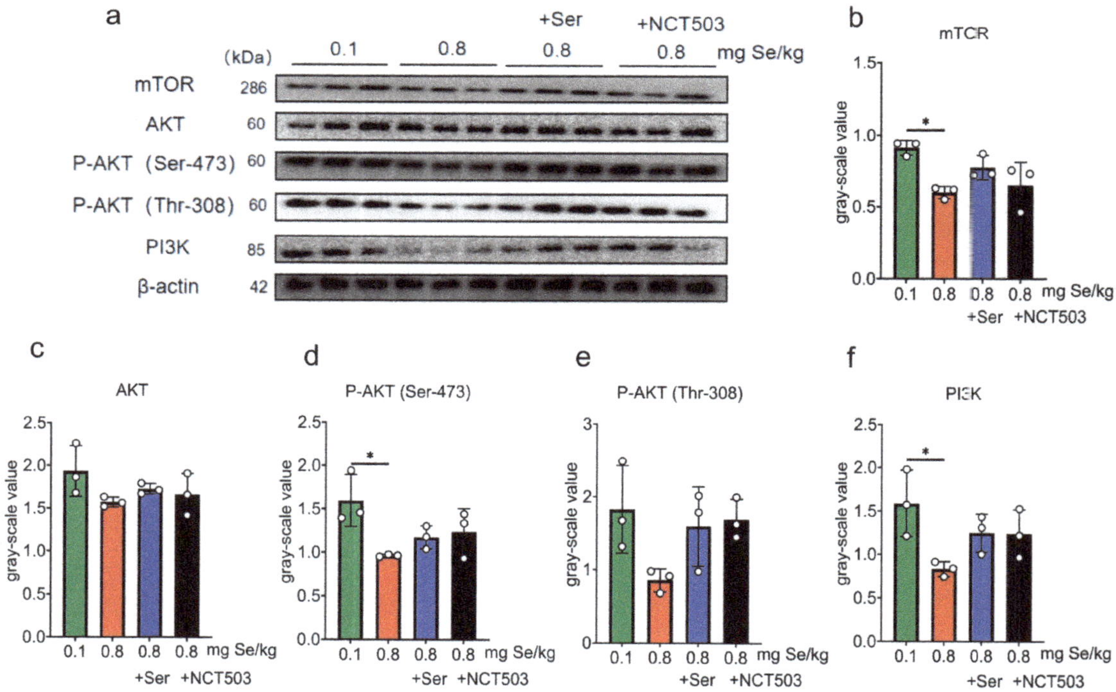

Figure 8. Effects of 0.1, 0.8 mg Se/kg, and Ser or the NCT503 intervention group on the PI3K-AKT-mTOR pathway in mice muscle. (**a**) WB images. (**b–f**) Pathway grayscale analysis (Mean ± SD, n = 3, * $p < 0.05$; two-way ANOVA). While Ser and NCT503 supplementation slightly increased Akt/mTOR pathway markers in muscle, these changes were not significant.

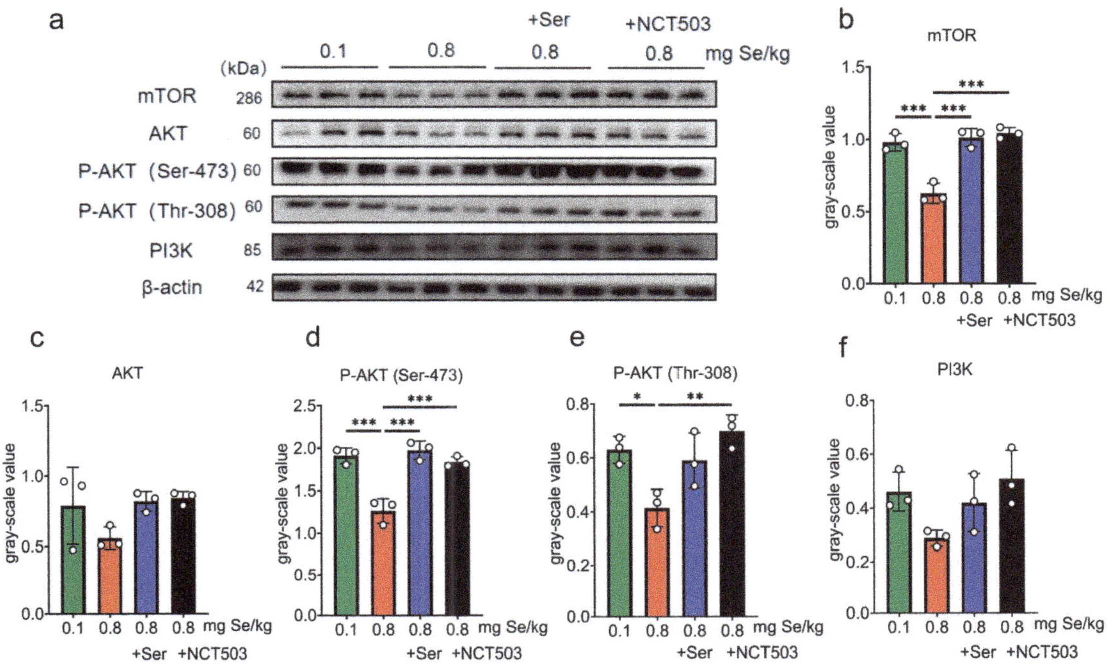

Figure 9. Effects of 0.1, 0.8 mg Se/kg, and Ser or the NCT503 intervention group on the PI3K-AKT-mTOR pathway in mice muscle pancreas. (**a**) WB images. (**b**–**f**) Pathway grayscale analysis (Mean ± SD, n = 3, * $p < 0.05$, ** $p < 0.01$, *** $p < 0.001$; two-way ANOVA). Both Ser and NCT503 supplementation restored Akt/mTOR signaling in the pancreas, with significant increases in mTOR and phosphorylated Akt levels compared to the high-Se group.

4. Discussion

At present, IR models have been developed through natural feeding with high-Se fodder in animals such as pigs, rats, mice, and chickens. Recently, we successfully re-established the high-Se-induced IR model in C57BL/6J mice fed with 0.4 mg Se/kg diet for 4 months based on the research [7]. In addition to the same occurrence of IR, we observed for the first time changes in the expressions of enzymes related to serine synthesis and metabolism [14].

Given the substantial evidence that excessive selenium intake beyond physiological needs raises the risk of diabetes in individuals, it mainly comes from two intervention cohort studies of selenium supplementation to prevent cancer in North America, and the total daily average selenium intake of subjects in the two cohort studies is 330 μg per day. In this study, the selenium content in the high selenium feed given to C57BL/6J mice increased from 0.4 mgSe/kg (equivalent to a daily selenium intake of 200 μg for adults) to 0.8 mgSe/kg (equivalent to a daily selenium intake of 400 μg for adults).

Excessive selenium intake (0.8 mg Se/kg) significantly disrupted glucose homeostasis, as evidenced by elevated fasting blood glucose levels, increased insulin secretion, impaired glucose tolerance, and reduced insulin sensitivity (Figures 2b–d and 3a). Notably, mice in the high-Se group exhibited a significantly greater final body weight compared to the two intervention groups, while the high-Se +serine group showed the lowest body weight among all groups (Figure 2a). This unexpected observation suggests a complex interaction between selenium and serine in energy metabolism. The specific mechanisms underlying this weight reduction remain to be elucidated. Additionally, selenium concentrations in plasma and tissues, as well as plasma serine levels, were markedly elevated in the high-Se group relative to the adequate-Se group (Figure 3c,d), implying systemic selenium accumulation under high-Se conditions.

Consistent with prior studies [14], we observed a pronounced upregulation of GPX1, SELENOP, and SELENON across the liver, muscle, and pancreas in mice exposed to a high-Se diet (Figures 4–6). These selenoproteins play pivotal roles in redox homeostasis, and their coordinated upregulation underscores the cellular need to counteract Se-induced oxidative damage. Importantly, serine supplementation enhanced the expression of GPX1 and SELENOP in the liver and SELENON in muscle, suggesting a synergistic interaction between serine and selenium in augmenting antioxidant defenses. This finding aligns with our previous research [12] and highlights serine's potential as a metabolic modulator in the context of selenium exposure.

PHGDH, the first rate-limiting enzyme in the SSP, is high-expressed in various metabolic disorders, including cancer and glucose metabolism [24–26], to produce serine supplying one-carbon unit for the synthesis of nucleotide to meet the need of tumor cell growth. In this study, the protein expression and enzyme activity of PHGDH were significantly increased in the high-Se group and were inhibited by exogenous serine (Figures 3e, 4d and 6c). The content of serine decreased for the high-Se +NCT-503 group (Figure 3c). We observed that NCT-503 did not suppress PHGDH protein expression in the liver, muscle, or pancreas (Figures 4d, 5d and 6c), but significantly inhibited PHGDH enzyme activity (Figure 3e). NCT503 is designed as a specific inhibitor targeting the active site of PHGDH, by directly binding to the active center of PHGDH, without reducing its expression through changes in protein stability or degradation rate [27]. Studies reported that NCT-503 inhibited PHGDH enzyme activity without affecting PHGDH protein expression [20,28,29], which aligns with the experimental results we observed.

Our study found that high-Se conditions significantly upregulated key enzymes involved in the methionine and folate cycles, including SHMT1 in the liver and pancreas (Figures 3e and 5d), MTHFR in the liver and muscle (Figures 4f and 5f), and MS in the liver, muscle, and pancreas (Figures 4g, 5g and 6e). These results were consistent with our previous observations that endogenous serine synthesis through SSP contributes to methyl group supply, facilitating SAM regeneration and subsequent selenium detoxification [14]. As Figure 10 shows, serine's dual role in redox balance and one-carbon metabolism underscores its central importance in mitigating selenium toxicity [30]. By providing one-carbon units through tetrahydrofolate intermediates, serine replenishes SAM, supports methylation reactions, and alleviates Se-induced oxidative stress. Additionally, serine enhances antioxidant defenses by promoting GSH synthesis via the transsulfuration pathway [31]. Interestingly, the observed upregulation of MS and SHMT1 was significantly inhibited by exogenous serine or NCT-503 (Figures 4g, 5g and 6d), which reveals that serine supplementation not only mitigates SSP overactivation but also restores methionine and folate cycle functions, alleviates metabolic burdens, and reduces selenium toxicity. Notably, pharmacological inhibition of PHGDH with NCT-503 achieves similar effects, further supporting SSP as a promising therapeutic target in managing selenium-induced metabolic dysfunction.

As we discussed in a previous study [14], Se-induced metabolic stress activates the SSP through upregulation of the rate-limiting enzyme PHGDH, leading to increased serine synthesis. However, excessive selenium consumption may place a substantial metabolic burden on redox balance. The activation of the PI3K-AKT-mTOR pathway is important for glucose intake [32–34]. Interestingly, the regulation of PHGDH and mTOR under high-Se stress follows distinct and independent pathways (Figure 11). While mTOR activity is attenuated by AMPK in response to energy and oxidative stress, SSP activation via PHGDH upregulation is primarily driven by ATF4 and FOXO1 [35]. As observed in this study, high-Se levels significantly downregulated phosphorylation of AKT at Ser473 and Thr308 (Figures 7d, 8d and 9d,e), diminished mTOR expression (Figures 8b and 9b), and reduced PI3K activity (Figure 8f), collectively indicating compromised pathway functionality. Supplementation with exogenous serine or NCT-503 enhanced the expressions of mTOR in the liver and pancreas (Figures 7b and 9b and P-AKT in the pancreas (Figure 9d,e), which implied alleviating SSP overactivation and restoring PI3K-AKT-mTOR pathway activity.

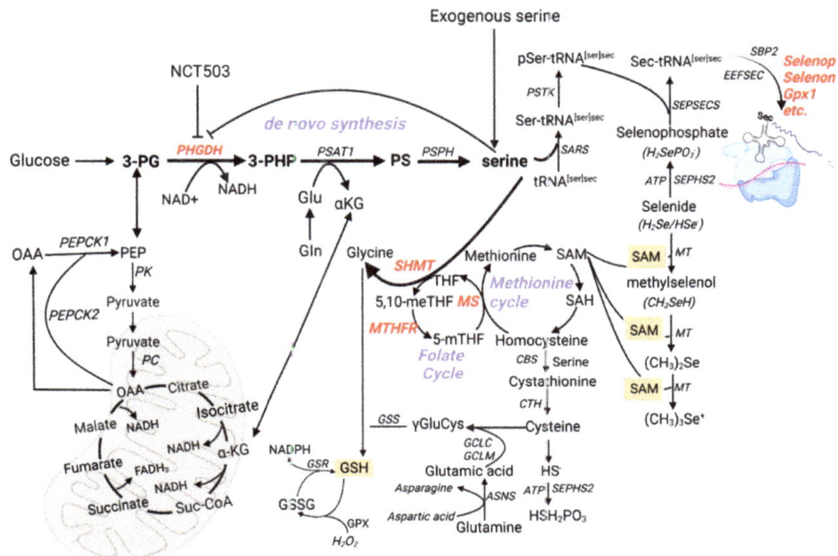

Figure 10. The SSP supports selenium detoxification and metabolic balance. The SSP plays a pivotal role in maintaining redox balance, supporting methylation reactions, and facilitating selenium detoxification under high selenium conditions. Increased PHGDH expression drives serine production, replenishing SAM for methylation and promoting GSH synthesis to combat oxidative stress. Excessive SSP activation burdens the methionine and folate cycles, depleting SAM and disrupting methylation homeostasis. Serine supplementation alleviates these effects by restoring one-carbon metabolism and enhancing selenium detoxification. Similarly, pharmacological inhibition of PHGDH (e.g., NCT-503) reduces SSP overactivation, highlighting its potential as a therapeutic target in Se-induced metabolic dysregulation.

The dose of serine in this study is 240 mg/kg body weight, which is also close to previous studies, such as the reported 280 mg/kg dose that ameliorated diabetic symptoms in murine models [36]. In healthy adults (average body weight 70 kg), the no-observed-adverse-effect-level (NOAEL) for L-serine is 12 g/day, corresponding to a daily intake of 171 mg/kg body weight [37]. According to the US FDA, L-serine, as a food additive, is considered safe when not exceeding 8.4% of total dietary protein (67.2 mg/kg body weight). For specific conditions (e.g., diabetes) or high-demand scenarios, L-serine supplementation can reach up to 30 g/day, equal to 429 mg/kg body weight [38]. Future studies should focus on characterizing the dose–response curve for serine supplementation, particularly at lower doses, to identify the minimal effective dose. Additionally, investigations should explore the appropriate equivalent dosing for humans and evaluate its safety and efficacy in clinical settings. Such research will be essential for refining dietary and therapeutic guidelines for serine use in mitigating excess Se-induced glucose metabolic dysregulation.

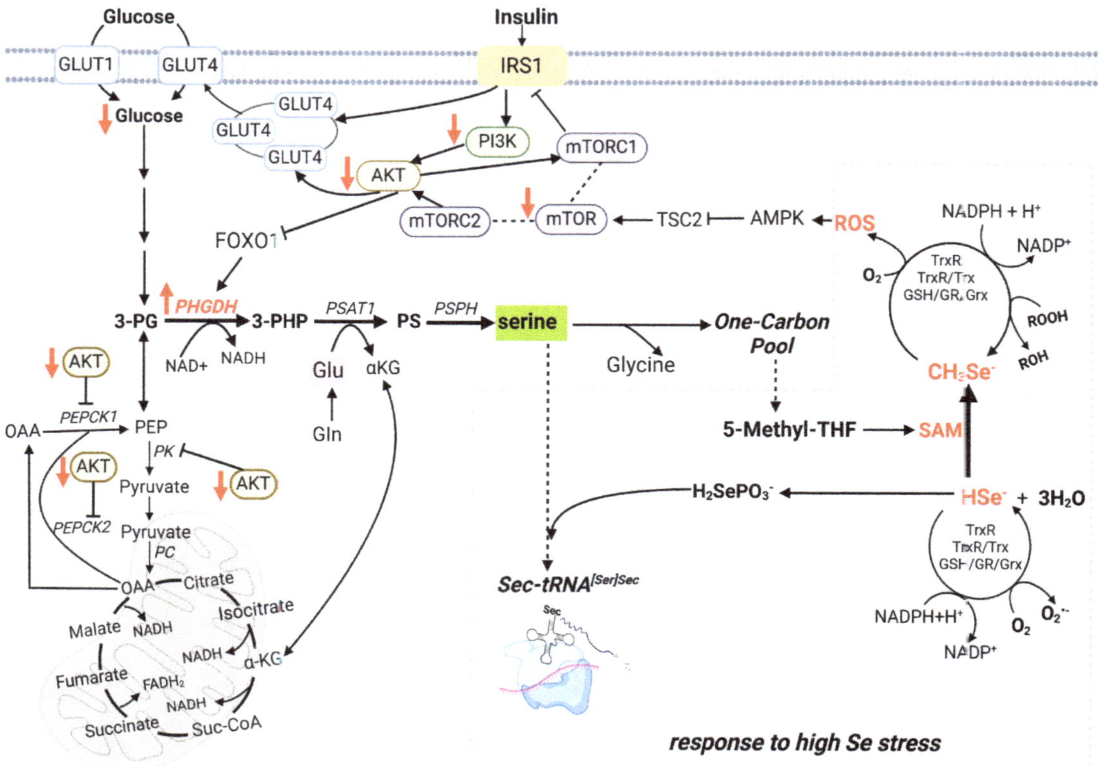

Figure 11. Integration of mTOR signaling, oxidative stress, and IR. The figure delineates the intricate mechanisms by which mTOR signaling integrates oxidative stress, energy homeostasis, and insulin sensitivity. Oxidative stress activates AMPK, which inhibits mTORC1 via TSC2 phosphorylation and suppresses Rheb, a key mTOR activator. Reduced mTOR signaling impairs AKT activation, disrupting GLUT4 translocation and diminishing glucose uptake. Concurrently, impaired AKT fails to suppress FOXO1 nuclear activity, leading to enhanced gluconeogenesis through the upregulation of key enzymes like PEPCK. Elevated oxidative stress and inflammation further aggravate IR by activating pathways, inducing aberrant IRS1 phosphorylation, and reducing insulin receptor sensitivity. These combined effects underscore the centrality of mTOR in maintaining redox balance, metabolic stability, and insulin signaling integrity.

Despite the comprehensive investigation of high Se-induced IR and the mitigating effects of serine supplementation and PHGDH inhibition, several limitations remain in this study. First, our findings are based on C57BL/6J mice, which may not fully capture interspecies differences or directly translate to human physiology. Second, while the 5-month duration of selenium exposure and serine supplementation was sufficient for experimental observations, it does not reflect chronic long-term exposure scenarios in humans. Furthermore, additional studies involving a broader range of animal models and a detailed exploration of serine dosage are required to better understand its application and establish effective and safe dosing guidelines for potential human use.

5. Conclusions

In this study, we provide further evidence for the pivotal role of the SSP in high Se-induced glucose metabolic dysfunction. Our study observed the effects of serine supplementation to mitigate SSP overactivation, modulate methionine and folate cycles, and reactivate the PI3K-AKT-mTOR signaling pathway. By evaluating serine as both a dietary and therapeutic agent, this study could establish a foundation for translational applications in addressing metabolic disorders related to excessive selenium exposure, including IR and diabetes.

Supplementary Materials: The following supporting information can be downloaded at: https://www.mdpi.com/article/10.3390/nu17020311/s1, Table S1: Glucose levels, body weight, OGTT, and ITT area under the curve (AUC) results; Table S2: Changes in plasma biochemical markers (insulin, homocysteine and serine); Table S3: Selenium Levels in Mouse Plasma, Liver, Muscle, and Pancreas (μg/kg); Table S4: PHGDH Enzyme Activity in Mouse Liver, Muscle, and Pancreas (U/g); Table S5: Analysis of Western Blot Grayscale Values in Mouse Liver; Table S6: Analysis of Western Blot Grayscale Values in Mouse Muscle; Table S7: Analysis of Western Blot Grayscale Values in Mouse Pancreas.

Author Contributions: S.Z. conducted the experiments, performed statistical analyses, created the figures, and wrote the manuscript; Q.W. revised the paper. J.W., M.Z., F.H., L.S., and Y.L. contributed to the experiments and writing. Z.H. critically reviewed the manuscript. All authors have read and agreed to the published version of the manuscript.

Funding: This work was funded by the National Natural Science Foundation of China (Grant Nos. 81973048, 81741032, and 81372989), the Public Health Emergency Project Nutrition Health and Healthy Diet Campaign (No. 102393220020070000012).

Institutional Review Board Statement: This study was conducted in accordance with the guidelines of the Helsinki Declaration and was approved by the Ethics Committee of the National Institute of Nutrition and Health (protocol code 2020-NINH-IACUC-033, approved on 23 September 2020). The animals were housed in the animal facility of the National Institute for Occupational Health and Poison Control, Chinese Center for Disease Control and Prevention. Appropriate measures, including the use of anesthesia, environmental enrichment, and humane handling, were taken to minimize pain, suffering, and distress during the experimental procedures. The sample size is based on previous studies in the same field to ensure consistency and reliability of the results, while minimizing the use of animals according to the 3R (replace, reduce, improve) principle.

Informed Consent Statement: Not applicable.

Data Availability Statement: The data presented in this study are experimental data generated during the research. These experimental data are available in the Supplementary Materials.

Conflicts of Interest: The authors have no relevant financial or non-financial interests to disclose.

References

1. Huang, X.; Yang, X.; Zhang, M.; Li, T.; Zhu, K.; Dong, Y.; Lei, X.; Yu, Z.; Lv, C.; Huang, J. SELENOI Functions as a Key Modulator of Ferroptosis Pathway in Colitis and Colorectal Cancer. *Adv. Sci.* **2024**, *11*, e2404073. [CrossRef] [PubMed]
2. Begum, M.; Choubey, M.; Tirumalasetty, M.B.; Arbee, S.; Mohib, M.M.; Wahiduzzaman, M.; Mamun, M.A.; Uddin, M.B.; Mohiuddin, M.S. Adiponectin: A Promising Target for the Treatment of Diabetes and Its Complications. *Life* **2023**, *13*, 2213. [CrossRef] [PubMed]
3. McClung, J.P.; Roneker, C.A.; Mu, W.; Lisk, D.J.; Langlais, P.; Liu, F.; Lei, X.G. Development of insulin resistance and obesity in mice overexpressing cellular glutathione peroxidase. *Proc. Natl. Acad. Sci. USA* **2004**, *101*, 8852–8857. [CrossRef] [PubMed]
4. Yan, X.; Pepper, M.P.; Vatamaniuk, M.Z.; Roneker, C.A.; Li, L.; Lei, X.G. Dietary selenium deficiency partially rescues type 2 diabetes-like phenotypes of glutathione peroxidase-1-overexpressing male mice. *J. Nutr.* **2012**, *142*, 1975–1982. [CrossRef]
5. Misu, H.; Takamura, T.; Takayama, H.; Hayashi, H.; Matsuzawa-Nagata, N.; Kurita, S.; Ishikura, K.; Ando, H.; Takeshita, Y.; Ota, T.; et al. A liver-derived secretory protein, selenoprotein P, causes insulin resistance. *Cell Metab.* **2010**, *12*, 483–495. [CrossRef] [PubMed]
6. Mita, Y.; Nakayama, K.; Inari, S.; Nishito, Y.; Yoshioka, Y.; Sakai, N.; Sotani, K.; Nagamura, T.; Kuzuhara, Y.; Inagaki, K.; et al. Selenoprotein P-neutralizing antibodies improve insulin secretion and glucose sensitivity in type 2 diabetes mouse models. *Nat. Commun.* **2017**, *8*, 1658. [CrossRef]

7. Zhou, J.; Huang, K.; Lei, X.G. Selenium and diabetes--evidence from animal studies. *Free Radic. Biol. Med.* **2013**, *65*, 1548–1556. [CrossRef] [PubMed]
8. Labunskyy, V.M.; Lee, B.C.; Handy, D.E.; Loscalzo, J.; Hatfield, D.L.; Gladyshev, V.N. Both Maximal Expression of Selenoproteins and Selenoprotein Deficiency Can Promote Development of Type 2 Diabetes-Like Phenotype in Mice. *Antioxid. Redox Signal.* **2011**, *14*, 2327–2336. [CrossRef]
9. Zeng, M.-S.; Li, X.; Liu, Y.; Zhao, H.; Zhou, J.-C.; Li, K.; Huang, J.-Q.; Sun, L.-H.; Tang, J.-Y.; Xia, X.-J.; et al. A high-selenium diet induces insulin resistance in gestating rats and their offspring. *Free Radic. Biol. Med.* **2012**, *52*, 1335–1342. [CrossRef]
10. Lei, X.G.; Cheng, W.-H.; McClung, J.P. Metabolic regulation and function of glutathione peroxidase-1. *Annu. Rev. Nutr.* **2007**, *27*, 41–61. [CrossRef] [PubMed]
11. Huang, J.-Q.; Zhou, J.-C.; Wu, Y.-Y.; Ren, F.-Z.; Lei, X.G. Role of glutathione peroxidase 1 in glucose and lipid metabolism-related diseases. *Free Radic. Biol. Med.* **2018**, *127*, 108–115. [CrossRef]
12. Lennicke, C.; Cochemé, H.M. Redox regulation of the insulin signalling pathway. *Redox Biol.* **2021**, *42*, 101964. [CrossRef]
13. Wang, Q.; Sun, L.-C.; Liu, Y.-Q.; Lu, J.-X.; Han, F.; Huang, Z.-W. The Synergistic Effect of Serine with Selenocompounds on the Expression of SelP and GPx in HepG2 Cells. *Biol. Trace Elem. Res.* **2016**, *173*, 291–296. [CrossRef] [PubMed]
14. Liu, Y.; Wang, J.; Wang, Q.; Han, F.; Shi, L.; Han, C.; Huang, Z.; Xu, L. Effects of insufficient serine on health and selenoprotein expression in rats and their offspring. *Front. Nutr.* **2022**, *9*, 1012362. [CrossRef]
15. Wang, Q.; Wang, J.; Zhang, X.; Liu, Y.; Han, F.; Xiang, X.; Guo, Y.; Huang, Z.W. Increased Expression of PHGDH Under High-Selenium Stress In Vivo. *Biol. Trace Elem. Res.* **2024**, *202*, 5145–5156. [CrossRef] [PubMed]
16. Chen, W.; Yu, X.; Wu, Y.; Tang, J.; Yu, Q.; Lv, X.; Zha, Z.; Hu, B.; Li, X.; Chen, J.; et al. The SESAME complex regulates cell senescence through the generation of acetyl-CoA. *Nat. Metab.* **2021**, *3*, 983–1000. [CrossRef] [PubMed]
17. Hoffman, J.L. Selenite toxicity, depletion of liver S-adenosylmethionine, and inactivation of methionine adenosyltransferase. *Arch. Biochem. Biophys.* **1977**, *179*, 136–140. [CrossRef] [PubMed]
18. Maddocks, O.D.; Labuschagne, C.F.; Adams, P.D.; Vousden, K.H. Serine Metabolism Supports the Methionine Cycle and DNA/RNA Methylation through De Novo ATP Synthesis in Cancer Cells. *Mol. Cell.* **2016**, *61*, 210–221. [CrossRef] [PubMed]
19. Ye, L.; Sun, Y.; Jiang, Z.; Wang, G. L-Serine, an Endogenous Amino Acid, Is a Potential Neuroprotective Agent for Neurological Disease and Injury. *Front. Mol. Neurosci.* **2021**, *14*, 726665. [CrossRef]
20. Pacold, M.E.; Brimacombe, K.R.; Chan, S.H.; Rohde, J.M.; Lewis, C.A.; Swier, L.J.; Possemato, R.; Chen, W.W.; Sullivan, L.B.; Fiske, B.P.; et al. A PHGDH inhibitor reveals coordination of serine synthesis and one-carbon unit fate. *Nat. Chem. Biol.* **2016**, *12*, 452–458. [CrossRef]
21. McGuinness, O.P.; Ayala, J.E.; Laughlin, M.R.; Wasserman, D.H. NIH experiment in centralized mouse phenotyping: The Vanderbilt experience and recommendations for evaluating glucose homeostasis in the mouse. *Am. J. Physiol. Endocrinol. Metab.* **2009**, *297*, E849–E855. [CrossRef] [PubMed]
22. da Silva, I.J.; Lavorante, A.F.; Paim, A.P.; da Silva, M.J. Microwave-assisted digestion employing diluted nitric acid for mineral determination in rice by ICP OES. *Food Chem.* **2020**, *319*, 126435. [CrossRef]
23. Verity, N.; Ulm, B.; Pham, K.; Evangelista, B.; Borgon, R. Demonstrating core molecular biology principles using GST-GFP in a semester-long laboratory course. *Biochem. Mol. Biol. Educ.* **2022**, *50*, 55–64. [CrossRef] [PubMed]
24. Locasale, J.W.; Grassian, A.R.; Melman, T.; Lyssiotis, C.A.; Mattaini, K.R.; Bass, A.J.; Heffron, G.; Metallo, C.M.; Muranen, T.; Sharfi, H.; et al. Phosphoglycerate dehydrogenase diverts glycolytic flux and contributes to oncogenesis. *Nat. Genet.* **2011**, *43*, 869–874. [CrossRef] [PubMed]
25. Lee, C.M.; Hwang, Y.; Kim, M.; Park, Y.-C.; Kim, H.; Fang, S. PHGDH: A novel therapeutic target in cancer. *Exp. Mol. Med.* **2024**, *56*, 1513–1522. [CrossRef] [PubMed]
26. Okabe, K.; Usui, I.; Yaku, K.; Hirabayashi, Y.; Tobe, K.; Nakagawa, T. Deletion of PHGDH in adipocytes improves glucose intolerance in diet-induced obese mice. *Biochem. Biophys. Res. Commun.* **2018**, *504*, 309–314. [CrossRef] [PubMed]
27. Rohde, J.M.; Brimacombe, K.R.; Liu, L.; Pacold, M.E.; Yasgar, A.; Cheff, D.M.; Lee, T.D.; Rai, G.; Baljinnyam, B.; Li, Z.; et al. Discovery and optimization of piperazine-1-thiourea-based human phosphoglycerate dehydrogenase inhibitors. *Bioorganic Med. Chem.* **2018**, *26*, 1727–1739. [CrossRef]
28. Buqué, A.; Galluzzi, L.; Montrose, D.C. Targeting Serine in Cancer: Is Two Better Than One? *Trends Cancer* **2021**, *7*, 668–670. [CrossRef]
29. Spillier, Q.; Frédérick, R. Phosphoglycerate dehydrogenase (PHGDH) inhibitors: A comprehensive review 2015–2020. *Expert Opin. Ther. Pat.* **2021**, *31*, 597–608. [CrossRef]
30. Wu, D.; Zhang, K.; Khan, F.A.; Pandupuspitasari, N.S.; Guan, K.; Sun, F.; Huang, C. A comprehensive review on signaling attributes of serine and serine metabolism in health and disease. *Int. J. Biol. Macromol.* **2024**, *260 Pt 2*, 129607. [CrossRef]
31. Zhang, J.; Zou, S.; Fang, L. Metabolic reprogramming in colorectal cancer: Regulatory networks and therapy. *Cell Biosci.* **2023**, *13*, 25. [CrossRef]

32. Ramasubbu, K.; Rajeswari, V.D. Impairment of insulin signaling pathway PI3K/Akt/mTOR and insulin resistance induced AGEs on diabetes mellitus and neurodegenerative diseases: A perspective review. *Mol. Cell. Biochem.* **2023**, *478*, 1307–1324. [CrossRef] [PubMed]
33. Lu, X.; Xie, Q.; Pan, X.; Zhang, R.; Zhang, X.; Peng, G.; Zhang, Y.; Shen, S.; Tong, N. Type 2 diabetes mellitus in adults: Pathogenesis, prevention and therapy. *Signal Transduct. Target. Ther.* **2024**, *9*, 262. [CrossRef] [PubMed]
34. Barroso, E.; Jurado-Aguilar, J.; Wahli, W.; Palomer, X.; Vázquez-Carrera, M. Increased hepatic gluconeogenesis and type 2 diabetes mellitus. *Trends Endocrinol. Metab.* **2024**, *35*, 1062–1077. [CrossRef] [PubMed]
35. Jin, N.; Bi, A.; Lan, X.; Xu, J.; Wang, X.; Liu, Y.; Wang, T.; Tang, S.; Zeng, H.; Chen, Z.; et al. Identification of metabolic vulnerabilities of receptor tyrosine kinases-driven cancer. *Nat. Commun.* **2019**, *10*, 2701. [CrossRef] [PubMed]
36. Langroudi, F.E.; Narani, M.S.; Kheirollahi, A.; Vatannejad, A.; Shokrpoor, S.; Alizadeh, S. Effect of L-serine on oxidative stress markers in the kidney of streptozotocin-induced diabetic mice. *Amino Acids* **2023**, *55*, 799–806. [CrossRef] [PubMed]
37. Miura, N.; Matsumoto, H.; Cynober, L.; Stover, P.J.; Elango, R.; Kadowaki, M.; Bier, D.M.; Smriga, M. Subchronic Tolerance Trials of Graded Oral Supplementation with Phenylalanine or Serine in Healthy Adults. *Nutrients* **2021**, *13*, 1976. [CrossRef]
38. Holm, L.J.; Buschard, K. L-serine: A neglected amino acid with a potential therapeutic role in diabetes. *APMIS Acta Pathol. Microbiol. Et Immunol. Scand.* **2019**, *127*, 655–659. [CrossRef] [PubMed]

nutrients

MDPI

Article

Mediation Effect of Oxidative Stress on Association Between Selenium Intake and Cognition in American Adults

Jia-Meng Li, Ya-Zhi Bai, Quan-Ying Liu and Shuang-Qing Zhang *

National Institute for Nutrition and Health, Chinese Center for Disease Control and Prevention, 27 Nanwei Road, Beijing 100050, China; ljmchinacdc@163.com (J.-M.L.); yzbaichinacdc@163.com (Y.-Z.B.); liuqychinacdc@163.com (Q.-Y.L.)

* Correspondence: zhangsq@ninh.chinacdc.cn or zhangshq@hotmail.com; Tel.: +86-10-66237226

Abstract: Objectives: Dementia affects millions of aged people globally and mainly results from oxidative stress. Selenium shows beneficial effects on dementia however it remains elusive for the mediation effect of oxidative stress on the association between selenium and cognition. The present study firstly investigated the potential mediation role of oxidative stress on the relationship of selenium and cognition. Methods: A total of 2154 adults aged 60 years and older from the National Health and Nutrition Examination Survey 2011–2014 were selected for the study. Weighted multivariate linear regression, weighted logistic regression, and mediation effect analysis were employed to investigate the association among selenium intake, cognition, and oxidative stress. Results: Selenium intake was positively associated with cognition, albumin, and vitamin D, negatively associated with uric acid, and exhibited no correlation with gamma glutamyl transpeptidase (GGT). Cognition was positively correlated with albumin and vitamin D, negatively related to GGT, and had no association with uric acid. Albumin and vitamin D significantly mediated the relationship between selenium intake and cognition, and the mediation proportion values of albumin and vitamin D were 3.85% and 8.02%, respectively. Conclusions: For the first time, our findings demonstrated that higher selenium intake decreased cognitive impairment and oxidative stress levels. Moreover, the relationship between selenium intake and cognition was mediated by oxidative stress

Keywords: selenium intake; cognition; oxidative stress; mediation effect; National Health and Nutrition Examination Survey

1. Introduction

Dementia, the seventh leading cause of death and one of the major reasons for disability and dependency, affects about 55.2 million people worldwide, and its global cost is projected to grow from $1.3 trillion in 2019 to $1.7 trillion in 2030 [1]. Therefore, it is imperative for the prevention and treatment of dementia. Despite decades of extensive research, effective clinical therapies for dementia remain limited [2]. Fortunately, several studies have indicated that selenium shows beneficial effects on dementia [3].

Selenium, an essential micronutrient for humans provided by various foods, is distributed throughout the body, particularly in the brain [4]. Compared to zinc and copper, selenium attenuated the negative association of co-exposure to arsenic, cadmium, and lead with cognitive function [5]. It plays crucial roles in cognition [1], including antioxidation [6], anti-inflammation [4], modulation of the levels of metals such as zinc and copper [7], enhancement of synaptic plasticity, inactivation of ferroptosis, and regulation of de novo synthesis of L-serine and PI3K/mTOR/GSK3 [4]. Selenium deficiency has been recognized as an important contributing factor to dementia due to its detrimental effects on humans [8]. However, inconsistent results were observed in human studies on the association between selenium and cognition. A cross-sectional study conducted on 1681 Americans over 65 years old found higher cognitive scores in individuals with higher selenium intakes [9];

however, no association was observed between plasma selenium and cognition in 154 Australian adults aged 60 years and older [10]. Therefore, it is necessary to analyze the association between selenium intake and cognition.

Oxidative stress results from the imbalance between reactive oxygen species (ROS) and antioxidant defenses [11]. ROS inflicts damage upon neuronal cellular membranes, proteins, and deoxyribonucleic acid, impairs neuroelectric conduction and synaptic plasticity, and finally leads to dementia [12]. Albumin, gamma glutamyl transpeptidase (GGT), uric acid, and serum vitamin D are usually used as biomarkers of oxidative stress [13]. Although the association between these biomarkers and dietary fat intake had been disclosed [14], the relationship between these biomarkers and trace elements such as selenium has not been investigated. Therefore, these biomarkers are first employed to investigate the relationship between selenium intake and oxidative stress in our study. Mediation effect analysis decomposes the overall impact of exposure on outcomes into a direct effect and an indirect effect through a mediator variable, and its strength lies in the utilization of non-parametric test and the derivation of causality between variables. Some studies found the positive correlation between selenium intake and cognition using multiple linear regression or logistic regression [3,9]. To date, no study analyses the relationship between selenium intake and cognition through mediation effect analysis.

Therefore, for the first time, by virtue of oxidative stress biomarkers and mediation effect analysis, our study aimed to investigate the association between selenium intake and oxidative stress, as well as the association between selenium intake and cognition using the National Health and Nutrition Examination Survey (NHANES) 2011–2014. Our work might provide selenium as a valuable therapy option for the improvement of cognitive function.

2. Methods

2.1. Study Population

The NHANES represents a groundbreaking initiative that aims to evaluate the health and nutritional status of adults and children in the research program. The distinguishing aspect of this survey lies in its comprehensive approach, which integrates interviews and physical examinations. Each year, the survey examines a nationally representative sample comprising approximately 5000 individuals distributed in 15 counties. The National Center for Health Statistics Ethics Review Board approved the present study, and all participants signed informed consent forms. Additional ethics approval was not necessary because our research was based upon a secondary analysis. Our study utilized data from 19,931 people surveyed in the NHANES 2011–2014. Following the exclusion criteria in Figure 1, a total of 2154 participants were eligible for the analysis, in which 745 people took selenium supplementation.

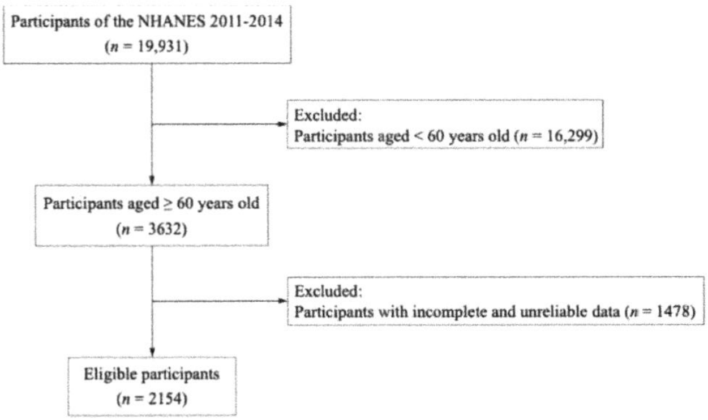

Figure 1. The selection process of the study participants.

2.2. Selenium Intake

Selenium intake was evaluated using two 24 h dietary recalls. Dietary recall interviews were conducted in person by trained diet interviewers fluent in Spanish and English. A Mobile Examination Center (MEC) was utilized to serve areas selected for inclusion in order to provide ease of access to participants. Interviewers that gathered participant information underwent a week-long training program to ensure proper technique and the following of protocol when interviewing participants. The first interview was collected in the MEC in person, and the second one was carried out by telephone 3–10 days later. Upon the completion of the in-person interview, measuring cups, spoons, a ruler, and a food model booklet containing two-dimensional drawings of the various measuring guides available in the MEC were given to participants for use in reporting food amounts during the telephone interview. The total selenium intake was calculated by the average selenium intake of two days of dietary selenium plus supplemental selenium.

2.3. Cognitive Function

The cognitive function assessment consisted of the following three parts: (1) the Consortium to Establish a Registry for Alzheimer's disease (CERAD), (2) the animal fluency test, and (3) the Digit Symbol Substitution test (DSST).

The CERAD word learning subtest was used to assess immediate and delayed recall of new linguistic information (the memory sub-domain) through three consecutive learning trials followed by a delayed recall session. In the learning experiment, participants were instructed to read aloud 10 unrelated words, 1 at a time. Immediately after word introduction, participants recalled as many words as possible. The sequence of 10 words was changed for each of 3 learning trials. The maximum possible score per trial was 10. In the NHANES, the words for the learning trials were displayed in large bold letters on a computer monitor. Participants who were unable to read due to literacy or visual impairment were asked to repeat each word after the interviewer had read it. Delayed word recall occurred after completion of the other two cognitive exercises (animal fluency and DSST) (approximately 8–10 min from the beginning of the word learning trial). The animal fluency test examined categorical language fluency. Participants were asked to name as many animals as possible in one minute. Each named animal will receive one point. In the NHANES, participants were first asked to name three items of clothing, another verbal fluency category, as a practice test. Participants who were unable to name three items of clothing did not proceed with the animal fluency exercise. The DSST is a performance module of the Wechsler Adult Intelligence Scale used to assess subjects' processing speed, continuous attention, and working memory. Participants taking part in the DSST had two minutes to copy the relevant symbol number adjacent to the 133 boxes. The score was the total number of correct matches. Sample practice tests were conducted before participants began the main test. In the NHANES, participants who were unable to correctly match symbols to numbers on their own during pre-test practice did not continue. The total scores of the three parts were used as the general cognitive function score, the lowest quartile was considered as cognitive impairment, and the rest was normal cognition [15].

2.4. Oxidative Stress Biomarkers

Beckman Coulter UniCel DxC800 (Beckman Coulter, Fullerton, CA, USA) used various methods, including a bichromatic digital endpoint method for albumin measurement, an enzymatic rate method to determine GGT, and a timed endpoint method for the measurement of uric acid. Vitamin D, the sum of 25-hydroxyvitamin D2 and 25-hydroxyvitamin D3, was detected by ultra-high performance liquid chromatography-tandem mass spectrometry.

2.5. Study Covariates

Covariates were chosen mainly based on factors associated with cognitive function in the previous studies [16,17]. In our study, covariates included age (≥60 years), gender (male and female), race (Mexican American, other Hispanic, Non-Hispanic White,

Non-Hispanic Black, and other race), educational level (less than high school, high school, and more than high school), and marital status (married/living with a partner, widowed/divorced/separated, and never married), poverty/income ratio (PIR) ($\leq$1.3, 1.3–4.0, >4.0) [18], and body mass index (BMI) (underweight: <18.5 kg/m^2; normal: 18.5–24.9 kg/m^2; overweight: 25–29.9 kg/m^2; obesity: $\geq$30 kg/m^2) [19]. Participants were defined as "drinkers" if they had at least 12 alcohol drinks in the previous year [14]. Smoking at least 100 cigarettes in life was defined as "smokers" [15]. Additionally, the history of diseases (hypertension, diabetes mellitus, coronary heart disease, and stroke) was included [3].

2.6. Statistical Analysis

Statistical analysis was conducted using SAS 9.4 (SAS Institute Inc., Cary, NC, USA) and R version 4.3.1. Continuous variables are presented as the mean $\pm$ standard deviation (SD) and categorical variables are expressed as cases (n) and percentages (%). Differences among means were analyzed by Rao-Scott χ^2 test or ANOVA.

With selenium intake as an independent variable and oxidative stress as a dependent variable, weighted multivariate linear regression models were used to explore the association between selenium intake and oxidative stress. Weighted logistic regression models were employed to investigate the relationship between selenium intake and cognition, as well as oxidative stress and cognition. Three models were used in our study. Model 1 was a crude model not adjusted for potential confounding factors. Model 2 was adjusted for age, gender, race, educational level, and marital status. Model 3 was further adjusted for PIR, BMI, smoking, alcohol use, and comorbidities (diabetes, hypertension, stroke, and coronary heart disease).

The strategy of distribution-of-the-product was applied to detect the potential mediation role of oxidative stress in the association between selenium intake and cognitive function by checking (1) the association between selenium intake (the main determinant) and cognition (the outcome), adjusting age, gender, race, educational level, marital status, PIR, BMI, smoking status, drinking status, and diseases history (path c); (2) the association between selenium (the main determinant) and oxidative stress (the outcome), adjusting age, gender, race, educational level, marital status, PIR, BMI, smoking status, drinking status, and diseases history (path a); (3) the effect of selenium (the main determinant) on cognition (the outcome), making adjustment for the same covariates (path c'); and (4) the indirect effect (path a $\times$ path b). The R mediation package was used to evaluate the mediation effect of oxidative stress on the relationship between selenium intake and cognition. Mediation proportions and p-values were obtained after 1000 simulations using the quasi-Bayesian Monte Carlo method [20]. All statistical tests were two-sided, and $p < 0.05$ was regarded as statistically significant.

3. Results

3.1. General Characteristics of Participants

The characteristics of individuals categorized by cognition status are summarized in Table 1. There were significant differences between subjects with cognitive impairment and normal cognition in age, race, educational level, marital status, drinking, PIR, diabetes mellitus history, hypertension history, stroke history, and oxidative stress biomarkers ($p < 0.05$) but not in gender, smoking status, BMI, and coronary heart disease history ($p > 0.05$). In addition, selenium intakes in the normal cognition group were higher than those in the cognitive impairment group ($p < 0.01$).

Table 1. General characteristics of participants (n = 2154).

Characteristic	Cognitive Impairment		p
	Yes (n = 544)	No (n = 1610)	
Age, years [a]	73.57 ± 6.43	68.03 ± 6.31	<0.01
Gender [b]			0.80
Male	302 (47.77)	741 (46.95)	-
Female	242 (52.23)	869 (53.05)	-
Race [b]			<0.01
Mexican American	63 (7.19)	114 (2.58)	-
Other Hispanic	84 (9.92)	114 (2.52)	-
Non-Hispanic White	202 (60.95)	922 (83.74)	-
Non-Hispanic Black	172 (17.87)	310 (6.14)	-
Other Race	23 (4.08)	150 (5.03)	-
Education [b]			<0.01
Less than high school	259 (37.66)	219 (9.96)	-
High school	142 (30.43)	376 (20.65)	-
More than high school	143 (31.90)	1015 (69.39)	-
Marital status [b]			<0.01
Married or living with a partner	279 (55.90)	998 (69.14)	-
Widowed/separated/divorced	237 (40.19)	520 (27.08)	-
Never married	28 (3.91)	92 (3.79)	-
Smoker [b]			0.78
Yes	286 (50.16)	808 (49.12)	-
No	258 (49.84)	802 (50.88)	-
Drinker [b]			<0.01
Yes	347 (61.72)	1156 (75.73)	-
No	197 (38.28)	454 (24.27)	-
Income [b]			<0.01
PIR ≤ 1.3	258 (38.16)	335 (12.44)	-
PIR 1.3–4.0	225 (46.81)	734 (43.52)	-
PIR > 4.0	61 (15.03)	541 (44.04)	-
BMI, kg/m^2 [b]			0.10
Underweight: <18.5	13 (3.79)	20 (1.16)	-
Normal: 18.5–24.9	136 (25.39)	402 (25.62)	-
Overweight: 25–29.9	186 (35.94)	572 (35.78)	-
Obesity: ≥30	209 (34.87)	616 (37.43)	-
Diabetes mellitus [b]			<0.01
Yes	194 (32.54)	403 (20.06)	-
No	350 (67.46)	1207 (79.94)	-
Hypertension [b]			<0.01
Yes	382 (69.31)	963 (56.79)	-
No	162 (30.69)	647 (43.21)	-
Stroke [b]			<0.01
Yes	61 (10.68)	85 (4.97)	-
No	483 (89.32)	1525 (95.03)	-
Coronary heart disease [b]			0.05
Yes	68 (12.97)	138 (9.06)	-
No	476 (87.03)	1472 (90.94)	-
Dietary + Supplemental selenium intake, μg/d [a]	113.09 ± 53.80	134.67 ± 63.29	<0.01
GGT, U/L [a]	28.99 ± 42.51	23.75 ± 22.10	<0.01
Albumin, mg/mL [a]	4.12 ± 0.35	4.22 ± 0.27	<0.01
Uric acid, mg/dL [a]	5.68 ± 1.44	5.57 ± 1.44	<0.01
Vitamin D, nmol/L [a]	78.35 ± 32.81	84.30 ± 32.48	<0.01

[a] Continuous variables with a normal distribution were expressed as mean ± SD and p value was tested by ANOVA. [b] Categorical variables were expressed as the number of subjects (percentage) and p value was tested by the Rao-Scott χ^2 test. BMI: body mass index; PIR: poverty/income ratio; GGT: gamma glutamyl transpeptidase. "-" means blank.

3.2. Relationship Among Selenium Intake, Cognition, and Oxidative Stress

The relationship between selenium intake and cognition is presented in Table 2. The results of weighted logistic regression models showed that there was a statistically significant positive association between selenium intake and cognition in models 1, 2, and 3 ($p < 0.0001$).

Table 2. The relationship between selenium and cognition ($n = 2154$).

Variables	OR (95% CI)	p
Model 1	1.007 (1.004, 1.010)	<0.0001
Model 2	1.005 (1.002, 1.008)	0.0046
Model 3	1.004 (1.001, 1.007)	0.0191

Model 1: Unadjusted. Model 2: Adjusted for age, gender, race, marital status, and educational level. Model 3: Adjusted model 2 variables and family poverty/income ratio, body mass index, smoking, alcohol use and comorbidities (diabetes, hypertension, stroke, and coronary heart disease). CI: confidence interval; OR: odds ratio.

The relationship between oxidative stress and cognition is displayed in Table 3. The results of weighted logistic regression models showed that GGT was negatively correlated with cognition in all models ($p < 0.05$). Albumin was positively correlated with cognition in model 1 ($p = 0.0011$) and model 3 ($p = 0.0154$), and was negatively associated with cognition in model 2 ($p = 0.0084$). In all models, vitamin D was positively associated with cognition ($p < 0.05$). The association between uric acid and cognition was not found in all models ($p > 0.05$).

Table 3. The relationship between oxidative stress and cognition ($n = 2154$).

Variables	GGT		Albumin		Uric Acid		Vitamin D	
	OR (95% CI)	p	OR (95% CI)	p	OR (95% CI)	p	OR (95% CI)	p
Model 1	0.994 (0.990, 0.998)	<0.001	3.067 (1.621, 5.804)	0.001	0.952 (0.866, 1.046)	0.297	1.006 (1.002, 1.010)	0.005
Model 2	0.993 (0.988, 0.998)	0.014	0.854 (0.820, 0.889)	0.008	1.057 (0.941, 1.187)	0.339	1.006 (1.003, 1.010)	<0.001
Model 3	0.994 (0.988, 0.999)	0.030	2.073 (1.161, 3.701)	0.015	0.857 (0.823, 0.893)	0.236	1.005 (1.002, 1.009)	0.007

Model 1: Unadjusted. Model 2: Adjusted age, gender, race, marital status, and educational level. Model 3: Adjusted model 2 variables and family poverty/income ratio, body mass index, smoking, alcohol use, and comorbidities (diabetes, hypertension, stroke, and coronary heart disease). CI: confidence interval; GGT: gamma glutamyl transpeptidase.

The relationship between selenium intake and oxidative stress is exhibited in Table 4. The results of weighted multivariate linear regression models indicated that selenium intake was positively correlated with albumin and vitamin D ($p < 0.05$), and was negatively correlated with uric acid in all models ($p < 0.05$). No significant association was found between selenium intake and GGT in all models ($p > 0.05$).

Table 4. The relationship between selenium and oxidative stress ($n = 2154$).

Variables	Model 1		Model 2		Model 3	
	β (95% CI)	p	β (95% CI)	p	β (95% CI)	p
GGT	−0.0088 (−0.031, 0.013)	0.4153	−0.0145 (−0.0385, 0.0095)	0.2270	−0.0125 (−0.0385, 0.0134)	0.3319
Albumin	0.0005 (0.0003, 0.0008)	<0.0001	0.0004 (0.0002, 0.0006)	0.0019	0.0003 (0.0001, 0.0005)	0.0063
Uric acid	−0.0001 (−0.0015, 0.0014)	0.9272	−0.0018 (−0.0033, −0.0004)	0.0145	−0.0016 (−0.0030, −0.0002)	0.0246
Vitamin D	0.0129 (−0.0282, 0.0539)	0.5280	0.0356 (0.0001, 0.0710)	0.0491	0.0308 (−0.0002, 0.0618)	0.0514

Model 1: Unadjusted. Model 2: Adjusted age, gender, race, marital status, and educational level. Model 3: Adjusted model 2 variables and family poverty/income ratio, body mass index, smoking, alcohol use, and comorbidities (diabetes, hypertension, stroke, and coronary heart disease). CI: confidence interval; GGT: gamma glutamyl transpeptidase.

3.3. Mediation Effect of Oxidative Stress on Association Between Selenium Intake and Cognition

Based on the analysis among selenium intake, cognition, and oxidative stress, significant associations were chosen and the mediation was tested. Table 5 showed that after adjusting the controlled variables, albumin significantly mediated the link between selenium intake and cognition (proportion mediated, 3.85%; indirect effect, 2.61×10^{-4} [6.30×10^{-6}–5.31×10^{-4}], $p < 0.01$), and the direct effect of selenium intake on cognition in the absence of the mediation of albumin was also significant ($p < 0.01$). The relationship between selenium intake and cognition was significantly mediated by vitamin D (proportion mediated, 8.02%; indirect effect, 5.36×10^{-5} [1.63×10^{-5}–9.90×10^{-5}], $p < 0.01$), as shown in Figure 2.

Table 5. The mediation effect of oxidative stress on the association between selenium and cognition ($n = 2154$).

Variables	Estimate	95% CI		p
		Lower	Upper	
Albumin				
Total effect	6.43×10^{-4}	3.70×10^{-4}	9.15×10^{-4}	<0.01
Direct effect	6.16×10^{-4}	3.45×10^{-4}	8.81×10^{-4}	<0.01
Indirect effect	2.61×10^{-4}	6.30×10^{-6}	5.31×10^{-4}	<0.01
Proportion mediated	3.85×10^{-2}	9.27×10^{-3}	9.30×10^{-2}	<0.01
Vitamin D				
Total effect	6.60×10^{-4}	3.90×10^{-4}	9.22×10^{-4}	<0.01
Direct effect	6.05×10^{-4}	3.40×10^{-4}	8.69×10^{-4}	<0.01
Indirect effect	5.36×10^{-5}	1.63×10^{-5}	9.90×10^{-5}	<0.01
Proportion mediated	8.02×10^{-2}	2.35×10^{-2}	17.53×10^{-2}	<0.01

CI: confidence interval.

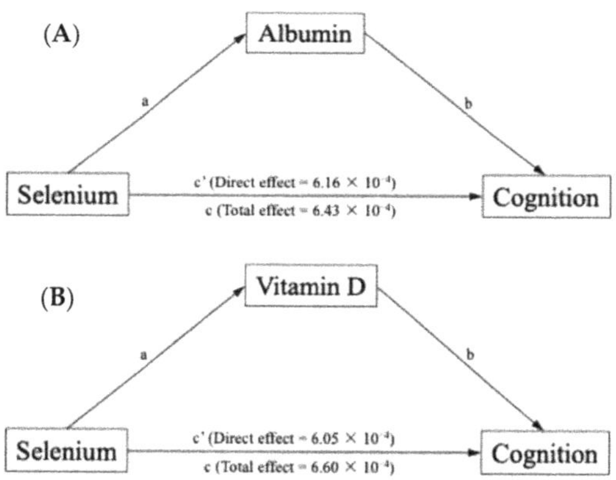

Figure 2. Indirect effects of selenium on cognition in mediation design. (**A**) The mediation effect of albumin on the association between selenium and cognition. (**B**) The mediation effect of vitamin D on the association between selenium and cognition.

4. Discussion

Our study investigated the relationship between selenium intake and cognition, and the results showed that subjects with higher selenium intake had a lower risk of cognitive impairment, which aligned with the previous reports [3,9,16,21]. However, a randomized clinical trial reported no relationship between selenium intake and cognition, and the discrepancy may be ascribed to only male subjects involved in the study [22].

Our results also disclosed that oxidative stress was a risk factor for cognitive impairment. Albumin was positively correlated with cognition in our research, which was consistent with the previous study [13,23,24]. Due to its distinct biological structure, specifically the cysteine residues at position 34, albumin had the potential to alleviate excessive oxidative stress caused by inflammation in aging neuronal cells, so it was regarded as an important biomarker for the evaluation of cognitive impairment in aging brains [23,25].

Participants with a higher vitamin D level exhibited better cognitive performance, which was in line with the previous results [26,27]. Vitamin D played a fundamental role in the maintenance of normal physiological function of neurons through the regulation of neuroprotective factors and/or oxidative stress [28]. Participants with a lower GGT level had higher cognition, which was in agreement with the previous reports [13,14,29]. GGT served a crucial function in maintaining the transport of glutathione into cells, thereby favoring cellular protective antioxidant capability [30]. Although there were similar uric acid levels in our research (5.6 mg/dL) and previous reports (5.3 [31] and 5.2 [32] mg/dL), the level of uric acid in our investigation was not correlated with cognitive performance, which was inconsistent with previous cross-sectional studies [31,32], possibly due to the Chinese population that participated in their reports. The inconsistency reminded us that the characteristics of the study population should be fully considered. If the study involved people from different regions, it was necessary to conduct an in-depth analysis of the various characteristics of the population. Oxidative stress level was significantly increased in the brain tissues of patients with cognitive impairment [33,34], and our results strongly supported the negative association between oxidative stress and cognition.

For the first time, we discovered that selenium intake was negatively associated with oxidative stress. Selenium was a key factor in maintaining human health by clearing free radicals, improving the activity of antioxidant enzymes, and inhibiting oxidative stress reactions [35,36]. Additionally, our present study firstly proposed that albumin and vitamin D had an incomplete mediated effect (i.e., the indirect effect was small and the direct effect was significant) on the association between selenium intake and cognition, suggesting that additional pathways (such as anti-inflammation and ferroptosis) besides antioxidation could be involved in the regulation of effects of selenium on cognition [4,37].

This study had several strengths. Firstly, it was the first study to investigate the relationship between selenium intake and cognition mediated by oxidative stress. Secondly, large national representative samples of elderly adults in the US increased the extrapolation of the results. Thirdly, all information were derived from highly valid NHANES records, and potential confounding factors were controlled in data analysis. However, several limitations also existed in this study. First, the NHANES was a cross-sectional study, which did not allow causal inferences. Second, dietary selenium data were self-reported, which might be subject to recall bias. Third, socioeconomic status and lifestyle factors may have important impacts on selenium intake and cognitive function. People with higher socioeconomic status and/or healthy lifestyles have opportunities to consume more selenium.

5. Conclusions

For the first time, our findings demonstrated that higher selenium intake decreased cognitive impairment and oxidative stress levels. Moreover, the relationship between selenium intake and cognition was mediated by oxidative stress.

Author Contributions: Original draft preparation, J.-M.L.; review and editing, Y.-Z.B. and Q.-Y.L.; conceptualization, review, editing, and supervision, S.-Q.Z. All authors have read and agreed to the published version of the manuscript.

Funding: This work was financially supported by the National Natural Science Foundation of China (grant number 82073855).

Institutional Review Board Statement: The NHANES was approved by the Institutional Review Committee of the National Centre for Health Statistics. Due to the present study based on the secondary analysis, additional ethics approval was not required.

Informed Consent Statement: Written informed consent was obtained from all subjects involved in the study.

Data Availability Statement: Datasets are publicly available at https://www.cdc.gov/nchs/nhanes/index.htm (accessed in 2017). The data have not been previously presented orally or by poster at scientific meetings.

Conflicts of Interest: The authors declare no conflicts of interest.

Abbreviations

BMI	body mass index
CERAD	Consortium to Establish a Registry for Alzheimer's disease
DSST	Digit Symbol Substitution test
GGT	gamma glutamyl transpeptidase
NHANES	National Health and Nutrition Examination Survey
PIR	poverty/income ratio
ROS	reactive oxygen species

References

1. Li, J.M.; Bai, Y.Z.; Zhang, S.Q. Roles of selenium in cognition. *Int. J. Vitam. Nutr. Res.* **2024**, *94*, 323–324. [CrossRef] [PubMed]
2. Li, J.M.; Bai, Y.Z.; Zhang, S.Q. Advances and challenges in serine in the central nervous system: Physicochemistry, physiology, and pharmacology. *Metab. Brain Dis.* **2024**, *39*, 1637–1647. [CrossRef] [PubMed]
3. Li, S.; Sun, W.; Zhang, D. Association of zinc, iron, copper, and selenium intakes with low cognitive performance in older adults: A cross-sectional study from National Health and Nutrition Examination Survey (NHANES). *J. Alzheimers Dis.* **2019**, *72*, 1145–1157. [CrossRef] [PubMed]
4. Bai, Y.Z.; Zhang, Y.; Zhang, S.Q. New horizons for the role of selenium on cognitive function: Advances and challenges. *Metab. Brain Dis.* **2024**, *39*, 1255–1268. [CrossRef]
5. Cheng, B.J.; Sheng, J.; Wang, H.L.; Wang, Y.; Cao, H.J.; Li, X.D.; Zhou, T.T.; Meng, X.L.; Nie, H.H.; Wang, S.F.; et al. Selenium attenuates the association of co-exposure to arsenic, cadmium, and lead with cognitive function among Chinese community-dwelling older adults. *Environ. Sci. Pollut. Res. Int.* **2023**, *30*, 36377–36391. [CrossRef]
6. Zhang, S.Q.; Zhang, H.B.; Zhang, Y. Quantification of selenomethionine in plasma using UPLC-MS/MS after the oral administration of selenium-enriched yeast to rats. *Food Chem.* **2018**, *241*, 1–6. [CrossRef] [PubMed]
7. Bai, Y.Z.; Zhang, S.Q. Selenium and children's cognition. *Int. J. Vitam. Nutr. Res.* **2024**, *94*, 161–162. [CrossRef]
8. Alehagen, U.; Opstad, T.B.; Alexander, J.; Larsson, A.; Aaseth, J. Impact of selenium on biomarkers and clinical aspects related to ageing: A review. *Biomolecules* **2021**, *11*, 1478. [CrossRef]
9. Ferdous, K.A.; Knol, L.L.; Park, H.A. Association between selenium intake and cognitive function among older adults in the US: National Health and Nutrition Examination Surveys 2011–2014. *J. Nutr. Sci.* **2023**, *12*, e57. [CrossRef]
10. Cardoso, B.R.; Szymlek-Gay, E.A.; Roberts, B.R.; Formica, M.; Gianoudis, J.; O'Connell, S.; Nowson, C.A.; Daly, R.M. Selenium status is not associated with cognitive performance: A cross-sectional study in 154 older Australian adults. *Nutrients* **2018**, *10*, 1847. [CrossRef]
11. Li, J.; Pan, L.; Pan, W.; Li, N.; Tang, B. Recent progress of oxidative stress associated biomarker detection. *Chem. Commun.* **2023**, *59*, 7361–7374. [CrossRef] [PubMed]
12. Solovyev, N.D. Importance of selenium and selenoprotein for brain function: From antioxidant protection to neuronal signalling. *J. Inorg. Biochem.* **2015**, *153*, 1–12. [CrossRef] [PubMed]
13. Song, L.; Li, H.; Fu, X.; Cen, M.; Wu, J. Association of the oxidative balance score and cognitive function and the mediating role of oxidative stress: Evidence from the National Health and Nutrition Examination Survey (NHANES) 2011–2014. *J. Nutr.* **2023**, *153*, 1974–1983. [CrossRef]
14. Liu, D.; Zhou, L.; Yang, M.; McIntyre, R.S.; Cao, B. Oxidative stress mediates the association between dietary fat intake and cognition in US older adults. *Am. J. Geriatr. Psychiatry* **2022**, *30*, 761–773. [CrossRef] [PubMed]
15. Lu, K.; Liu, T.; Wu, X.; Zhong, J.; Ou, Z.; Wu, W. Association between serum iron, blood lead, cadmium, mercury, selenium, manganese and low cognitive performance in old adults from National Health and Nutrition Examination Survey (NHANES): A cross-sectional study. *Br. J. Nutr.* **2023**, *130*, 1743–1753. [CrossRef] [PubMed]
16. Wang, X.; Wang, H.; Zhang, F.; Cui, Y.; Zhang, D.; Shen, X. Threshold effects and interactive effects of total zinc and selenium intake on cognitive function in older adults. *Clin. Nutr. ESPEN* **2022**, *47*, 383–390. [CrossRef]
17. Chen, J.; Fang, S.; Cai, Z.; Zhao, Q.; Yang, N. Dietary serine intake is associated with cognitive function among US adults. *Food Funct.* **2024**, *15*, 3744–3751. [CrossRef] [PubMed]
18. Bai, Y.Z.; Gao, Y.X.; Zhang, S.Q. Identification of factors on blood selenium levels in the US adults: A cross-sectional study. *Nutrients* **2024**, *16*, 1734. [CrossRef] [PubMed]
19. Wu, Y.; Lei, S.; Li, D.; Li, Z.; Zhang, Y.; Guo, Y. Relationship of Klotho with cognition and dementia: Results from the NHANES 2011–2014 and Mendelian randomization study. *Transl. Psychiatry* **2023**, *13*, e337. [CrossRef] [PubMed]

20. Tingley, D.; Yamamoto, T.; Hirose, K.; Keele, L.; Imai, K. Mediation: R package for causal mediation analysis. *J. Stat. Softw.* **2014**, *59*, 1–38. [CrossRef]
21. Jiang, K.; Xie, C.; Li, Z.; Zeng, H.; Zhao, Y.; Shi, Z. Selenium intake and its interaction with iron intake are associated with cognitive functions in Chinese adults: A longitudinal study. *Nutrients* **2022**, *14*, 3005. [CrossRef] [PubMed]
22. Kryscio, R.J.; Abner, E.L.; Caban-Holt, A.; Lovell, M.; Goodman, P.; Darke, A.K.; Yee, M.; Crowley, J.; Schmitt, F.A. Association of antioxidant supplement use and dementia in the prevention of Alzheimer's Disease by vitamin E and selenium trial (PREADViSE). *JAMA Neurol.* **2017**, *74*, 567–573. [CrossRef] [PubMed]
23. Min, J.Y.; Ha, S.W.; Yang, S.H.; Kang, M.J.; Jeong, D.E.; Min, K.B.; Kim, B. Chronic status of serum albumin and cognitive function: A retrospective cohort study. *J. Clin. Med.* **2022**, *11*, 822. [CrossRef] [PubMed]
24. Hu, Y.; Lin, D.; Song, M.; Wu, D.; Zhang, Y.; Li, G.; Luo, H. Sex and race differences in the association of albumin with cognitive function in older adults. *Brain Behav.* **2024**, *14*, e3435. [CrossRef]
25. Anraku, M.; Chuang, V.T.; Maruyama, T.; Otagiri, M. Redox properties of serum albumin. *Biochim. Biophys. Acta* **2013**, *1830*, 5465–5472. [CrossRef] [PubMed]
26. Pavlovic, A.; Abel, K.; Barlow, C.E.; Farrell, S.W.; Weiner, M.; DeFina, L.F. The association between serum vitamin D level and cognitive function in older adults: Cooper center longitudinal study. *Prev. Med.* **2018**, *113*, 57–61. [CrossRef]
27. Yang, T.; Wang, H.; Xiong, Y.; Chen, C.; Duan, K.; Jia, J.; Ma, F. Vitamin D supplementation improves cognitive function through reducing oxidative stress regulated by telomere length in older adults with mild cognitive impairment: A 12-month randomized controlled trial. *J. Alzheimers Dis.* **2020**, *78*, 1509–1518. [CrossRef]
28. Gall, Z.; Szekely, O. Role of vitamin D in cognitive dysfunction: New molecular concepts and discrepancies between animal and human findings. *Nutrients* **2021**, *13*, 3672. [CrossRef]
29. Praetorius Bjork, M.; Johansson, B. Gamma-Glutamyltransferase (GGT) as a biomarker of cognitive decline at the end of life: Contrasting age and time to death trajectories. *Int. Psychogeriatr.* **2018**, *30*, 981–990. [CrossRef]
30. Yavuz, B.B.; Yavuz, B.; Halil, M.; Cankurtaran, M.; Ulger, Z.; Cankurtaran, E.S.; Aytemir, K.; Ariogul, S. Serum elevated gamma glutamyltransferase levels may be a marker for oxidative stress in Alzheimer's disease. *Int. Psychogeriatr.* **2008**, *20*, 815–823. [CrossRef]
31. Liu, M.; Wang, J.; Zeng, J.; He, Y. Relationship between serum uric acid level and mild cognitive impairment in Chinese community elderly. *BMC Neurol.* **2017**, *17*, e146. [CrossRef] [PubMed]
32. Xiu, S.; Zheng, Z.; Guan, S.; Zhang, J.; Ma, J.; Chan, P. Serum uric acid and impaired cognitive function in community-dwelling elderly in Beijing. *Neurosci. Lett.* **2017**, *637*, 182–187. [CrossRef] [PubMed]
33. Horvat, P.; Kubinova, R.; Pajak, A.; Tamosiunas, A.; Schottker, B.; Pikhart, H.; Peasey, A.; Kozela, M.; Jansen, E.; Singh-Manoux, A.; et al. Blood-based oxidative stress markers and cognitive performance in early old age: The HAPIEE study. *Dement. Geriatr. Cogn. Disord.* **2016**, *42*, 297–309. [CrossRef] [PubMed]
34. Hajjar, I.; Hayek, S.S.; Goldstein, F.C.; Martin, G.; Jones, D.P.; Quyyumi, A. Oxidative stress predicts cognitive decline with aging in healthy adults: An observational study. *J. Neuroinflamm.* **2018**, *15*, e17. [CrossRef] [PubMed]
35. Huang, J.; Xie, L.; Song, A.; Zhang, C. Selenium status and its antioxidant role in metabolic diseases. *Oxid. Med. Cell Longev.* **2022**, *2022*, e7009863. [CrossRef] [PubMed]
36. Kielczykowska, M.; Kocot, J.; Pazdzior, M.; Musik, I. Selenium—A fascinating antioxidant of protective properties. *Adv. Clin. Exp. Med.* **2018**, *27*, 245–255. [CrossRef]
37. Liang, X.; Xue, Z.; Zheng, Y.; Li, S.; Zhou, L.; Cao, L.; Zou, Y. Selenium supplementation enhanced the expression of selenoproteins in hippocampus and played a neuroprotective role in LPS-induced neuroinflammation. *Int. J. Biol. Macromol.* **2023**, *234*, e123740. [CrossRef]

nutrients

MDPI

Article

Nano-Selenium Modulates NF-κB/NLRP3 Pathway and Mitochondrial Dynamics to Attenuate Microplastic-Induced Liver Injury

Qi Shen, Yunjie Liu, Jiakui Li * and Donghai Zhou *

College of Veterinary Medicine, Huazhong Agricultural University, Wuhan 430070, China; sysq@webmail.hzau.edu.cn (Q.S.); 18282644072@163.com (Y.L.)
* Correspondence: lijk210@mail.hzau.edu.cn (J.L.); vetim@mail.hzau.edu.cn (D.Z.)

Abstract: Background: Microplastics (PS-MPs) are a new type of pollutant with definite hepatotoxicity. Selenium, on the other hand, has natural, protective effects on the liver. Objectives/Methods: The purpose of this experiment is to find out whether nano-selenium (SeNP) can alleviate liver damage caused by microplastics. Initially, we established through in vitro experiments that SeNP has the ability to enhance the growth of healthy mouse liver cells, while microplastics exhibit a harmful impact on normal mouse hepatocyte cell suspensions, leading to a decrease in cell count. Subsequently, through in vivo experiments on male ICR mice, we ascertained that SeNPs alleviated the detrimental impacts of PS-MPs on mouse liver. Results: SeNPs hinder the signaling pathway of NF-κB/NLRP3 inflammatory vesicles, which is crucial for reducing inflammation induced by PS-MPs. In terms of their mechanism, SeNPs hinder the abnormalities in mitochondrial fission, biogenesis, and fusion caused by PS-MPs and additionally enhance mitochondrial respiration. This enhancement is crucial in averting disorders in energy metabolism and inflammation. Conclusions: To summarize, the use of SeNPs hindered inflammation by regulating mitochondrial dynamics, thus relieving liver damage caused by PS-MPs in mice. The anticipated outcomes offer new research directions that can be referenced in terms of inflammatory injuries caused by PS-MPs.

Keywords: microplastics; nano-selenium; inflammation; mitochondrial dynamics; NF-κB/NLRP3 signaling pathway

1. Introduction

According to the relevant references, microplastics refer to plastic particles that have a diameter smaller than 5 mm [1–3]. Microplastics can be classified according to their sources, and as such can be divided into primary microplastics formed directly from industrial production and secondary microplastics produced by the decomposition of plastic-type waste [4,5]. In contrast, classification of microplastics can occur according to the polymer type, which includes polyethylene, polystyrene, polypropylene, polyethylene terephthalate, and polyvinyl chloride. As a novel environmental pollutant, microplastics have been found in rivers, oceans, the atmosphere, drinking water, and food sources around the world [6–8]. A variety of organisms can be exposed to microplastics through breathing, eating, and drinking, which accumulate in the organisms themselves and are passed up the food chain, so it is inevitable that humans will ingest microplastics [9]. The available references estimate that the amount of microplastics ingested by a person, through their digestive and respiratory tracts, to be between 74,000 and 121,000 microplastics over the course of a year [10]. Microplastic particles have been found in several organs of living organisms, posing serious health risks [11–14], while the accumulation of microplastics in the liver of mice has been widely reported [15–17].

In the body, the liver serves as the biggest gland involved in digestion and detoxification. The primary factors contributing to liver disease are drug toxicity, viral infections, and malnutrition. Chronic liver disease can be caused by a variety of factors, including hepatocellular injury, cell death, hypoxia, or irregular cellular metabolism, among which microplastic-induced hepatocellular injury due to oxidative stress in hepatocytes cannot be ignored. Patients with severe chronic liver disease may develop liver cancer or liver failure, or it may even result in death [18–20]. It has been demonstrated that PS-MPs activate the transcriptional machinery in the liver of Labrador dogs, leading to the enhanced expression of lipid-related genes [21]. PS-MP exposure significantly increased the inflammatory response in the liver, as demonstrated by the increased infiltration of Kupffer cells (KCs) and the increased expression of pro-inflammatory markers [22].

Selenium plays an important role in antioxidative stress and anti-inflammatory regulation and is regarded as a crucial micronutrient that is indispensable for human well-being [23]. Selenium was discovered by the chemist Betserius [24]. The necessity of Se for living organisms is due to the fact that it is a component of selenocysteine (Sec), found in various selenoproteins. Many selenoproteins have pronounced antioxidant activity, thereby playing a crucial role in the antioxidant defense of cells as well as the maintenance of cell redox homeostasis. The representative selenoprotein is GPx, which belongs to the antioxidant enzyme family and its active center is Sec. It mainly reduces hydrogen peroxide and lipid peroxides produced during metabolism by GSH and regulates the cellular microenvironment to realize the detoxification of the body. While excessive selenium can be harmful, the body needs a daily intake of small quantities of selenium to sustain physiological functions [25]. After being absorbed in the gut, selenium finally reaches the liver, which serves as the main site of selenium metabolism. It has also been shown that the liver takes up and absorbs selenium better than other tissues in order to utilize it [26]. Selenium provides the liver with a robust defense mechanism against hepatitis and aids during the prevention of fatty liver disease [27–29]. It should be noted that selenium exists in many forms, and SeNPs are made up of tiny selenium particles at the nanoscale that are more biologically active and less toxic than other forms of selenium [30,31]. Therefore, in this study, an animal model of nano-selenium antagonism induced by microplastic-induced liver injury was used as an example to simultaneously investigate the effects of microplastics and nano-selenium on mouse liver cells, so as to determine the specific mechanisms of nano-selenium and to propose new therapeutic targets against microplastics.

2. Materials and Methods

2.1. Microplastics

White powder PS-MPs, with a particle size of 5 μm, were purchased from Shuangfu Plasticising Trading Co (GuangZhou, China). The chemical nature of the PS-MPs was polystyrene and it was visually observed to be in the form of a powder; in order to make it mix uniformly during the liquid phase, the suspension of the PS-MPs was carried out in such a way to ensure they were dispersed uniformly in sterilized water using ultrasonic waves. Finally, the suspension containing the PS-MPs was stored at room temperature, protected from light and reconstituted weekly.

2.2. Nano-Selenium

After being mixed together, 1% Bacillus licheniformis, with OD600 = 0.5 and 20 mmol/L sodium selenite, was subjected to agitation in a shaker (180 r/min, 37 °C) for a duration of 4 days. Subsequently, the resulting mixture was centrifuged at a speed of 12,000 revolutions per minute, for a period of 20 min, in order to disintegrate the bacteria. After washing, the precipitate was ground in liquid nitrogen. The powdered substance was collected and rinsed three times using sterile, ultrapure water at a temperature of 4 °C, rotating at a speed of 4000 revolutions per minute, for a duration of 5 min. Following sonication for 15 min in an ice bath, the powder underwent three successive washes that were performed with 1.5 M Tris-HCl in 1% SDS (Ph = 8.3) at 4 °C and 12,000 rpm for 8 min. Subsequently, the next step also involved washing with sterile ultrapure water at 4 degrees Celsius and 10,000 rpm for 8 min. The cleaned sediment was reconstituted using sterile ultrapure water, followed by the addition of n-octanol in a volumetric specific suspension ratio of n-octanol of 2:1. It was mixed thoroughly and centrifuged at 4 °C, 12,000 r/min for 8 min. This washing process was repeated 4 times. Once a stable nano-suspension of nano-selenium was achieved, it was resuspended using an adequate quantity of sterile ultrapure water. After obtaining lyophilized nano-selenium, the liquid was discarded following a washing process, and the resulting precipitate was then stored at −80 °C for one day. The precipitate was then removed and freeze-dried in a freeze-dryer (−40 °C) for 72 h and finally stored at room temperature away from light.

2.3. Characterization of PS-MPs and SeNPs

A layer of conductive adhesive was glued onto the sample holder, and the freeze-dried lyophilized SeNP nanopowder or PS-MP powder was glued onto the conductive adhesive by gently picking a bit of it up with a toothpick. The unglued sample powder was removed with an ear wash ball, and the sample was placed into the sample chamber for evacuation, liquid nitrogen addition, and gold sprinkling. Then, a suitable area in the field of view was selected for spot analysis. Particle size and energy spectra of PS-MPs and SeNPs were determined using field emission electron microscopy (Techcomp, Shanghai, China).

The mixture of PS-MPs and sterile water and the mixture of SeNPs and sterile water were diluted to 50 mg/L and sonicated, followed by transfer to a zeta flow cell and a quartz cuvette cell (Malvern Panalytical, Malvern, UK) for characterization. The liquid-phase surface charge of PS-MPs and SeNPs was measured using zeta potential and a particle size analyzer (Malvern Panalytical, Malvern, UK).

2.4. In Vitro Experimental Design

Nano-selenium was mixed with deionized water in different ratios and sonicated to produce 0.5, 1, 2, 2.5, and 5 μmol/L solutions of nano-selenium. Microplastics were mixed with deionized water in different ratios and sonicated to produce 5, 50, 500, 1000, 1500 and 2000 μg/mL microplastic solutions. Normal mouse hepatocyte (NCTC1469) suspension was added to the proportionally configured medium containing 1 per cent horse serum and DMEM/HIGH dextros and incubated for 12 h in a constant-temperature (5% CO_2, 37 °C) incubator (Panasonic) suitable for the survival of mouse hepatocytes. When the cell density reached 6.4×10^4 per well in 6-well plates and 2.5×10^4 per well in 96-well plates the next step was to treat them with different concentrations of PS-MPs and SeNPs.

2.4.1. Culture of Mouse Hepatocytes

The cryopreservation tubes were removed from the liquid nitrogen and the cells were quickly thawed in a 37 °C water bath. As soon as the cells thawed, they were removed from the water bath and the outside of the cryopreservation tubes was quickly sterilized with an alcohol sprayer before placing them on an ultraclean bench. The thawed cell cryopreservation solution (1 mL) was pipetted into a 10 mL sterile EP tube, 4 mL of DMEM/HIGH GLUCOSE Complete Medium with 10% horse serum was added, and the mixture was centrifuged for 5 min at room temperature, 1000 r/min. After removing the supernatant, the precipitate was resuspended with 5 mL of DMEM/HIGH GLUCOSE Complete Medium with 10% horse serum. After it was mixed well, the cell suspension was added to T25 with a pipette gun and incubated at 37 °C under 5% CO_2. During the incubation process, the solution was changed over 2–3 d. After the cells were fully grown, the test was carried out.

2.4.2. Cell Growth Curve Determination

To ensure that cells exposed to microplastics and nano-sized selenium were in the equilibrium growth phase and normal, we measured the growth curves of hepatocytes. Hepatocytes (NCTC1469) in good growth condition were taken and digested with trypsinase, and the cells were resuspended by adding an appropriate amount of medium to prepare the suspension. After cell counting, the cell concentration was adjusted to (1~5) $\times 10^4$ cells/mL, and the cells were accurately inoculated into two 24-well plates with the same amount of cell suspension added to each well. Samples were taken at the time points of 0, 4, 12, 24, and 48 h, and the cells were counted with a biological inverted microscope (XZ-10, Mshot, Guangzhou, China) and a Watson hemocyte counter (177-112C, WATSON, Tokyo, Japan). Measurements at each time point were made three times and independent samples were taken in triplicate for cell number determination. Finally, taking the incubation time as the horizontal axis and the cell concentration as the vertical axis, the cell concentration obtained at each time point was marked on coordinate paper, and the cell growth curve was obtained by connecting each point to the line.

2.4.3. Effect of PS-MPs on Hepatocyte Proliferation

Hepatocytes were counted using a biological inverted microscope (177-112C, WATSON, Tokyo, Japan) and Watson's blood cell counter (Watson, Japan), and the cytosol was diluted in suspension to 10,000 cells/mL with DMEM/HIGH GLUCOSE Complete Medium with 10% horse serum. The bottom of the T25 bottles was observed with an inverted microscope and when the cells occupied 80–90% of the bottom area of the bottle, 10 μL of the cell suspension was withdrawn and placed in a 96-well plate. Subsequently, the culture was supplemented with 5 μm of PS-MPs at concentrations of 5, 50, 500, 1000, 1500, and 2000 μg/mL in the culture. Following prolonged incubation at a temperature of 37 °C for a duration of 6 h, 10 μL of CCK8 reagent was introduced into every well, and the incubation process was extended for an additional 2 h. Absorbance was measured at 450 nm using zymography (BGM LABTECH, Offenburg, Germany) and cell inhibition was determined from the data collected.

2.4.4. Effect of SeNPs on Hepatocyte Proliferation

Based on the number of cells, the cell suspension was diluted to a concentration of 10,000 cells per milliliter. A volume of 10 μL of the cell suspension was withdrawn and introduced into 96-well plates. The bottom of the T25 flasks was observed using an inverted microscope, and when the area occupied by the cells reached 80–90% of the bottom area, selenium nano-solutions at concentrations of 0.5, 1, 2, 2.5, and 5 μmol/L were added to the cultures. Following a 12 h incubation period at a temperature of 37 °C, 10 μL of CCK8 solution was introduced into every well and left to incubate for a duration of 2 h. The measurement of absorbance was adjusted to 450 nm with zymography (BGM LABTECH, Germany) and the rate of cell proliferation was determined using the acquired data. We performed three biological replicates.

2.4.5. ROS Detection

The ROS Assay Kit (Bioland Biologicals, Guangzhou, China) was used to detect ROS levels in liver NCTC1469 cells in real time. NCTC1469 cells were inoculated into 12-well plates. The NCTC1469 cells were wall-plated overnight and then divided into 4 groups with 3 wells per plate. They were blank group (Con), microplastic group with 100 μL of 1000 μg/mL PS-MPs added by a pipette gun, nano-selenium + microplastic group with 100 μL of 1000 μg/μL PS-MPs and 100 μL of 1 μmol/L SeNPs, and nano-selenium group with 100 μL of 1 μmol/L SeNPs. After 6 h of treatment, the groups were processed following the steps in the instruction manual and finally observed under an inverted fluorescence microscope (MF53, Guangzhou, China). Under the microscope, ROS emitted green fluorescence, and we quantified the extent of oxidative stress to determine whether ROS production was induced by converting each set of images into 8-bit images via ImageJ and then calculating gray values for the fluorescent areas.

2.5. *In Vivo Experimental Design*

All ICR mice studied were provided by Hunan Slaughter Jingda Laboratory Animal Co. Ltd. and housed at the Animal Experimentation Centre of the College of Animal Medicine, Huazhong Agricultural University, where this study complied with animal ethics requirements (SYxk2020-0084, WuHan, China). Thirty-six male mice (4 weeks old) were divided into six groups (n = 6), which were the control group, the low-dose PS-MP group (0.1 mg/kg/d MPs), the medium-dose PS-MP group (1 mg/kg/d MPs), the high-dose PS-MP group (10 mg/kg/d MPs), the group that was exposed to both PS-MPs and SeNPs (10 mg/kg/d MPs + 1 mg/kg/d SeNPs), and the nano-selenium group (1 mg/kg/d SeNPs). The low-dose PS-MP solution (20 mg/L), medium-dose PS-MP solution (200 mg/L), and high-dose PS-MP solution (2000 mg/L) were prepared with pure water and PS-MP powder before the experiment. Nano-selenium solution (200 mg/L) was prepared with pure water and nano-selenium powder. All animals were kept in the experimental animal house and were given sufficient food and water during the feeding period, which was 28 days. The mice were weighed weekly with a weighing scale and treated daily with PS-MP solution and SeNPs by gavage. After 28 days, all mice were euthanized by injection of 5% pentobarbital sodium (200 mg/kg). Blood samples were collected by cardiac puncture for biochemical analysis and liver tissue was extracted for subsequent experiments.

2.5.1. H&E Staining of Liver

The mouse liver tissue was preserved in a 4% solution of paraformaldehyde for 24 h, followed by removal, dehydration in alcohol, and immersion in melted paraffin, and after the paraffin had solidified, it was trimmed for easy observation. Then, 5 μm sections of liver tissue embedded in paraffin were stained with hematoxylin and eosin. To make the sections transparent, the stained sections were dehydrated using anhydrous ethanol and subsequently washed with xylene. Ultimately, transparent portions were affixed with neutral resin and examined using a biological microscope (Ningbo Sunyu Instruments Co., Ltd., Ningbo, China).

2.5.2. TEM Observation of Liver Sections

The mouse liver tissue was first treated with 2.5% glutaraldehyde in phosphate buffer for a duration of 12 h, followed by a subsequent 2 h fixation in 1% osmium acid. Additionally, the tissue samples underwent dehydration using a gradient of ethanol and were subsequently embedded in acetone. Samples were sectioned in an ultrathin sectioning machine. Finally, transmission electron microscope (TEM) images at different magnifications were taken under a transmission electron microscope (HITACHI, Tokyo, Japan).

2.5.3. Blood Biochemical Analysis

Centrifuge tubes containing blood samples were placed in a 37 °C water bath for 5 min to produce the serum adequately. The serum was then placed in a high-speed refrigerated centrifuge (Centrifuge 5424R, Hamburg, Germany) at 4 °C, set at 4000 r/min, and centrifuged for 10 min. The BS-240VET (Mindray Biologicals Ltd., Shenzhen, China) was used to test serum biochemical parameters such as serum aspartate transaminase (AST), alanine aminotransferase (ALT), alkaline phosphatase (ALP), total bilirubin (T-BIL), direct bilirubin (D-BIL) and total bile acids (TBAs).

2.5.4. Bone Densitometry Analysis

Mice were euthanized and placed in a bone densitometer (InAlyzer Republic, MEDIKORS, Suwon City, Republic of Korea) for measurement of bone mineral content (BMC), bone mineral density (BMD), fat content in tissue, and liver coefficient.

2.5.5. Measurement of Antioxidant Indicators

Mouse serum malondialdehyde (MDA) levels, catalase (CAT), superoxide dismutase (SOD), and glutathione (GSH) activities were measured by assay kits (Nanjing Jiancheng Institute of Biological Engineering, Nanjing, China).

2.5.6. Immunofluorescence Staining

Mouse paraffin sections were deparaffinized in xylene and washed with distilled water, then placed in a repair cassette with citrate antigen repair buffer (PH 6.0) in a microwave oven for antigen repair, after which they were washed with PBS (PH 7.4) buffer. After the sections were shaken dry, the sections were covered with 3% BSA and left for 30 min at room temperature. Next, ABclonal NLRP3 Rabbit pAb (A5652) and NFKB1 Rabbit pAb (A6667) as primary antibodies at a dilution of 1/200 were added dropwise to the sections and incubated at 4 °C overnight. After the sections were washed with PBS (PH 7.4), secondary antibody (iNOS Rabbit mAb (A3774)) at a dilution of 1/2000 was added dropwise to the sections, then they were incubated for 50 min at room temperature and covered with neutral gum, and, ultimately, the sections were scrutinized and pictures were taken with a fluorescent microscope.

2.5.7. Quantitative Real-Time Quantitative Fluorescence PCR

The RNA was extracted from liver using Trizol reagent (Accurate Biology, Changsha, China) followed the manufacturer's instructions. Then, the total RNA was reverse-transcribed into complementary DNA (cDNA) by referring to the reverse transcription kit instructions of Novizan (Nanjing, China). We used the reaction system of TSE202 2 × T5 Fast qPCR Mix (SYBR Green I) from Tsingke (Wuhan, China). An amount of 4 μL of cDNA was used in each qPCR reaction. The preincubation cycle ran at 95 °C once for 60 s, and the number of qPCR cycles was 40. The PCR analysis was conducted on the LightCycler96 (Roche) with the employment of QuantStudio™ 5 design and analysis software. The mRNA sequences of NF-κB, P-NF-κB, TNF-α, Cleaved Caspase1, Caspase1, NLRP3, IL-1β, DRP1, OPA1, MFN1, MFN2, PGC1-α, and SIRT1 were acquired from NCBI GeneBank. The primers were synthesized by Wuhan Tsingke Engineering. The calculation of relative gene expressions was performed by the method of $2^{-\triangle\triangle Ct}$ with the use of GAPDH as the internal reference gene.

2.5.8. Western Blotting Analysis

Total proteins were extracted from liver tissues using RIPA lysate (Bi-osharp, Beijing, China), protein concentrations were determined by the Kaumas protein assay reagent, and the samples used were diluted to the same concentration by 0.9% NaCl for subsequent experiments. Next, the extracted protein samples were separated by 10% SDS-PAGE electrophoresis and subsequently transferred onto PVDF membranes. The membranes were soaked for 2 h in a mixture of skimmed milk and buffered saline (TBST) made from Tris and NaCl. Afterward, the PVDF filters were left to incubate overnight at a temperature of 4 °C with primary antibodies, which were diluted according to the provided guidelines. On the following day, the membranes underwent three washes with TBST solution for a duration of 5 min each. The membranes were then incubated overnight at 4 °C in secondary antibody diluted 1:8000 in TBST. Then, they were washed again in TBST 5 times for 5 min each at the end of the incubation. Both ECL A and ECL B were mixed in medium proportions in shaded centrifuge tubes, and PVDF membranes were placed in full contact with them and used for signal detection using a chemiluminescence imaging system (Nuclear Cheng Technology Development Co., Wuhan, China). All primary antibodies (NF-κB (p65), NLRP3, TNF-α, Caspase1, Cleaved Caspase1, P-NF-κB (p65), IL-1β, GAPDH) used in this section were from Wanlei bio and the secondary antibody was HRP-conjugated goat anti-rabbit IgG (H + L) (AS014) purchased from ABclonal (Wuhan, China).

3. Statistical Analysis

Data are reported as mean ± standard error of the mean (SEM) unless stated otherwise. Analysis of variance (ANOVA) was used for more than 2 groups. A p-value less than 0.05 was considered statistically significant. Statistical analysis and graphs were generated using GraphPad Prism 9.5 software: *: $p < 0.05$, **: $p < 0.01$, ***: $p < 0.001$, ns, not statistically significant; p-values of groups compared with each other: #: $p < 0.05$,

##: $p < 0.01$, ###: $p < 0.001$, ns: not statistically significant. All experiments were performed in 3 technical replicates. n = 6 for mouse experiments, n = 3 for cell experiments.

4. Results

4.1. Characterization of PS-MPs and SeNPs

According to the data presented in Figure 1A, the PS-MPs exhibit an average particle size of 5 μm and have a subspherical shape when observed using SEM. With TEM (Figure 1B), the SeNPs exhibit an approximately spherical shape with an average particle size of about 200 nm. Energy spectral scans were acquired for PS-MPs containing elements (Figure 1C,E) and SeNPs (Figure 1F,D) using SEM. The system is deemed to be highly stable if the magnitude of the zeta potential is equal to or greater than 30 mV, suggesting the presence of both electrostatic repulsion and spatial potential resistance among the particles [32]. The values of both PS-MPs (Figure 1G) and SeNPs (Figure 1H) are quite high. Zeta potential is a measure of the strength of the mutual repulsion or attraction between particles, and the higher the absolute value of zeta potential (positive or negative), the more the repulsive force exceeds the attractive force, which resists aggregation, and thus the more the system of selenium nanoparticles and microplastic solutions is stabilized.

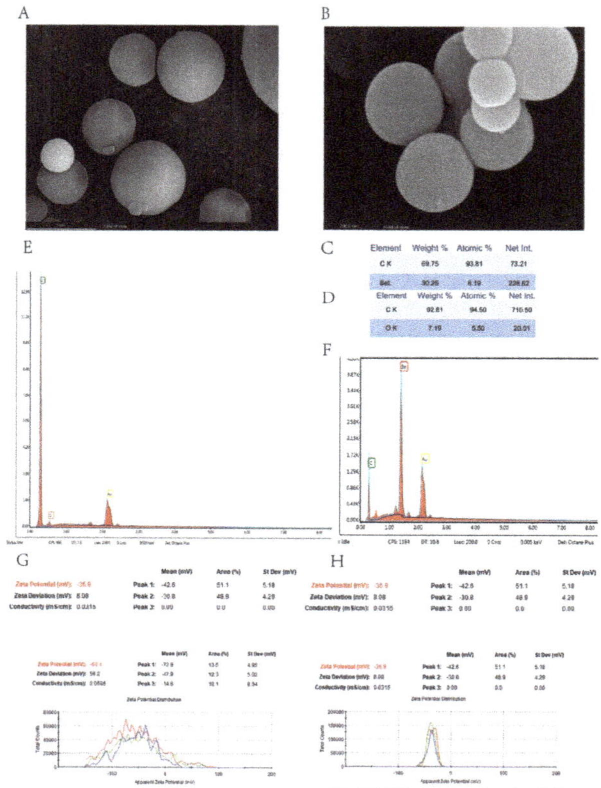

Figure 1. Characterization results of PS-MPs and SeNPs. (**A**) Scanning electron microscopy of PS-MPs. Scale bar, 5 μm. (**B**) Scanning electron microscopy of SeNPs. Scale bar, 200 nm. (**C**,**E**) EDS of PS-MPs. (**D**,**F**) EDS of SeNPs. (**G**) ζ-potential map of PS-MPs. (**H**) ζ-potential diagram of SeNPs.

4.2. *In Vitro Tests*

4.2.1. Determination of the Growth Curve of Normal Mouse Hepatocytes

Growth curves were established for normal mouse NCTC1469 hepatocytes. Cells were counted from the start of recovery and the total number of cells was then measured at 24 h, 48 h, and 72 h. Cells from 0–24 h were in the lag phase, 24–48 h cells were in the stationary phase, and 48–72 h cells were in the equilibrium phase. Therefore, NCTC1469 cells were cultured for 48 h before exposure to PS-MPs and SeNPs was performed (Figure 2A).

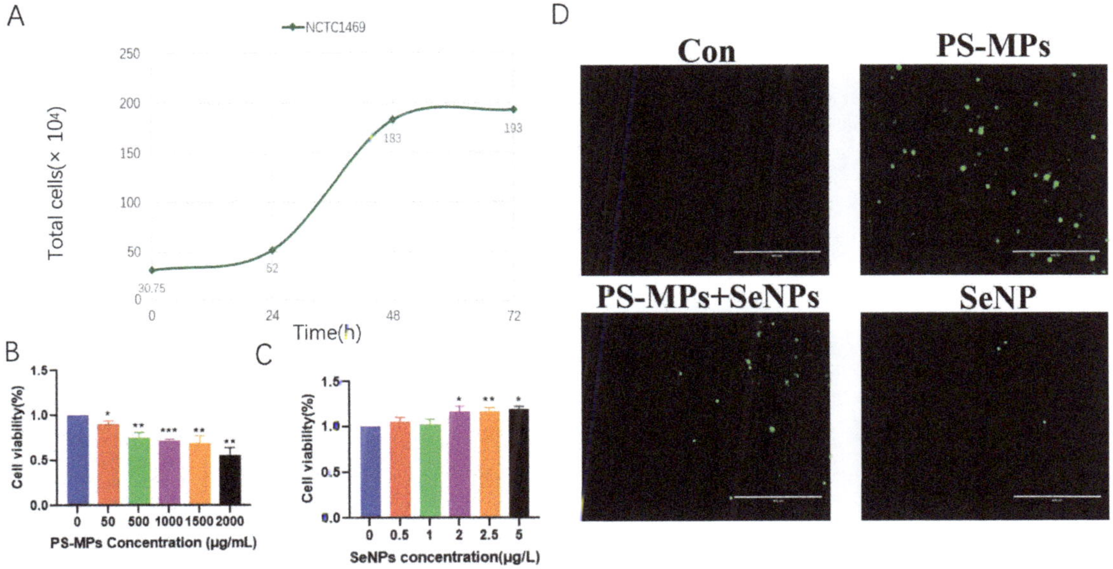

Figure 2. Effects of PS-MPs and SeNPs on mouse NCTC1469 hepatocyte lines. (**A**) Growth curves of normal mouse NCTC1469 hepatocyte cell suspensions, (**B**) cell survival rates after 6 h of action of different PS-MP concentrations (n = 3), (**C**) cell survival rates after 6 h of action of different SeNP concentrations (n = 3), (**D**) ROS fluorescence pictures of the groups. Scale bar, 400 μm. *: $p < 0.05$, **: $p < 0.01$, ***: $p < 0.001$.

4.2.2. Detection of Impact of PS-MPs on Hepatocytes by CCK8

Following a 6 h exposure to PS-MPs, the viability of normal NCTC1469 hepatocytes from mice gradually declined as the concentrations of PS-MPs increased. Specifically, the survival of cells was significantly inhibited at 50 μg/mL ($p < 0.05$), 500 μg/mL ($p < 0.01$), 1000 μg/mL ($p < 0.001$), 1500 μg/mL ($p < 0.01$), and 2000 μg/mL ($p < 0.01$) of PS-MPs. The concentration of PS-MPs chosen for the subsequent study (Figure 2B) was 2000 μg/mL, as it was nearer to the IC50.

4.2.3. Detection of Impact of SeNPs on Hepatocytes by CCK8

The impact of SeNPs on the viability of normal mouse NCTC1469 hepatocytes was observed for 6 h, as depicted in Figure 2C, at 0.5, 1, 2, 2.5, and 5 μmol/L. The findings indicated that small amounts of nano-selenium (0.5 μmol/L, 1 μmol/L) did not exhibit any harmful effect on mouse hepatocytes, and their cellular function was not notably distinct from that of the control group. However, when the concentration rose to 2 μmol/L, nano-selenium significantly stimulated the proliferation of hepatocytes ($p < 0.05$). Moreover, at a concentration of 2.5 μmol/L, their cellular activity displayed a highly significant difference ($p < 0.01$) compared to the control group.

4.2.4. Results of ROS Assay in Mouse Hepatocyte Suspensions

Upon examination of normal mouse NCTC1469 hepatocytes using a fluorescence microscope, it was observed that the fluorescence intensity of mouse hepatocytes in the PS-MP group exceeded that of the control group. However, the fluorescence intensity of the PS-MP + SeNP group was reduced after the addition of SeNPs. The fluorescence intensity of the control and SeNP groups was weaker (Figure 2D).

4.3. In Vivo Tests

4.3.1. Liver Dysfunction Induced by PS-MPs

Mouse serum biochemical parameters were measured in PS-MP-induced liver tissue (Figure 3A–F). The results of blood biochemical examinations indicated that the liver may be a target organ for PS-MPs. The expression levels of aspartate transaminase (AST), alanine aminotransferase (ALT), and serum alkaline phosphatase (ALP) were significantly higher in the exposed mice compared to the control. ALP was significantly increased in mice treated with 10 mg/mL of PS-MPs compared to the normal group. In addition, all other biochemical indices such as T-BIL, D-BIL, and TBA showed a significant increase in expression in a dose-dependent manner when compared to the control group.

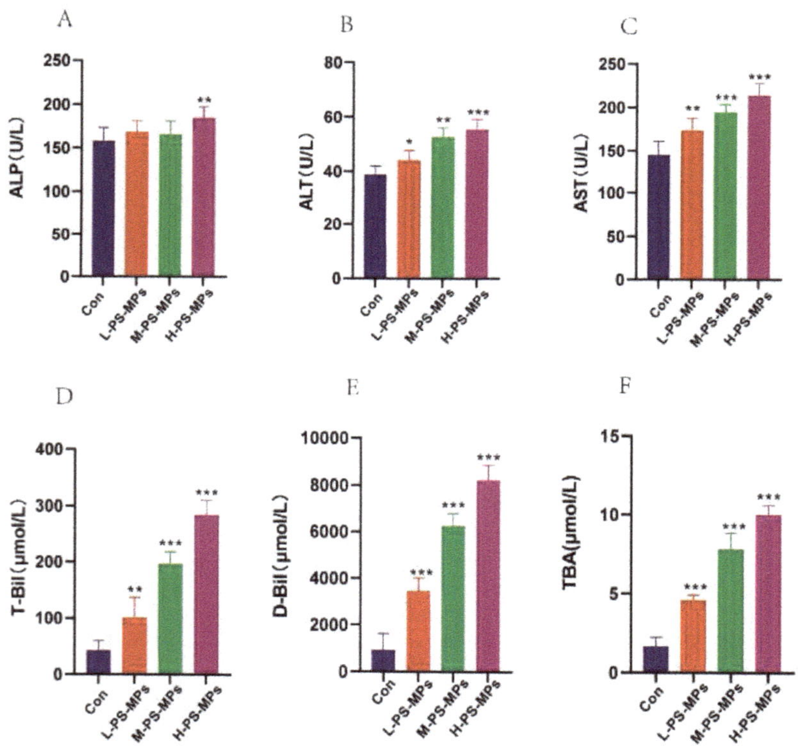

Figure 3. Effects of PS-MPs on biochemical indices in mice (n = 6). (**A**) Serum alkaline phosphatase (ALP), (**B**) serum alanine aminotransferase (ALT), (**C**) serum aspartate transaminase (AST), (**D**) total bilirubin (T-Bil), (**E**) direct bilirubin (D-Bil), (**F**) total bile acid (TBA). *: $p < 0.05$, **: $p < 0.01$, ***: $p < 0.001$.

4.3.2. Bone Densitometry Results in Mice

After being exposed for 28 days, the mice were euthanized and subjected to testing using a bone densitometer (Figure 4A). A notable variation in bone mineral content (BMC) was observed in the low-dose PS-MP group compared to the control group ($p < 0.05$), while the remaining groups did not show any significant difference (Figure 4C). On the other hand, there was no notable variation in BMD among the groups, which did not show any statistical significance (Figure 4D). Nonetheless, there existed a notable disparity in the lipid composition within the mouse tissues among all PS-MP groups and the control group, particularly in the high-dose PS-MP group (10 mg/kg/d) in comparison to the control group ($p < 0.001$) (Figure 4B). In addition, the liver ratios of mice in the high-dose PS-MP group (10 mg/kg/day) showed significant differences ($p < 0.01$) relative to the control group (Figure 4E). Hence, the high-dose category of PS-MPs (10 mg/kg/d) was employed as the ideal dosage of PS-MPs in Animal Experiment II for subsequent examinations.

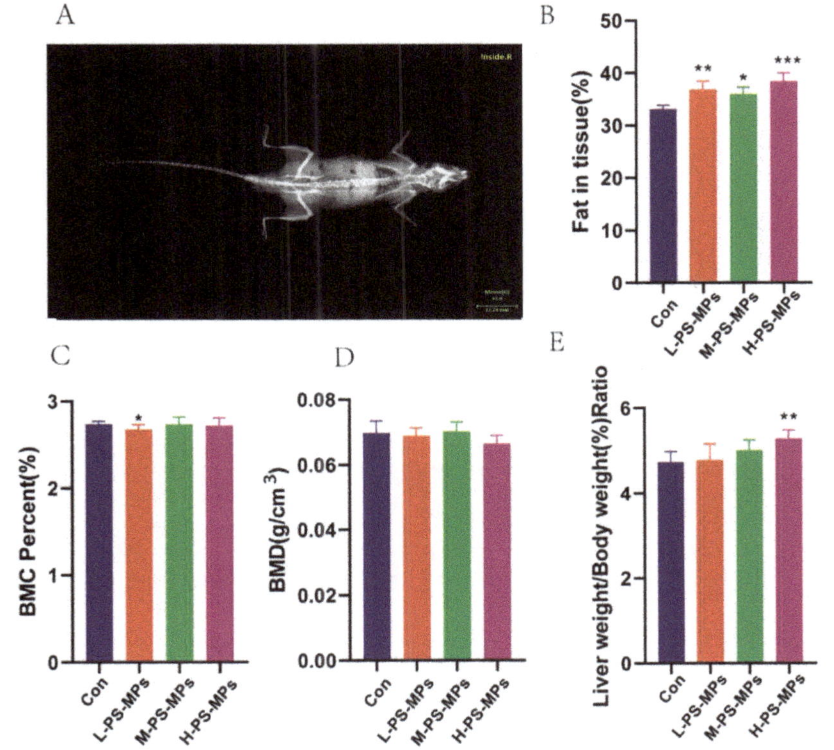

Figure 4. Radiographic images of mouse bone densitometry (n = 6). (**A**) Bone mineral density map (n = 6), (**B**) fat content in tissue (n = 6), (**C**) bone mineral content (BMC) (n = 6), (**D**) bone mineral density (BMD) (n = 6), (**E**) liver coefficient (n = 6). *: $p < 0.05$, **: $p < 0.01$, ***: $p < 0.001$.

4.3.3. SeNPs Reduce Liver Histopathological Abnormalities Caused by PS-MPs

In the H&E staining graphs of liver tissue sections (Figure 5A) it can be found that the control group showed normal hepatocyte morphology, with hepatocytes arranged in a spoke-like pattern, extending from the central vein in all directions, forming distinct hepatic cords. In contrast, the PS-MP group exhibited a markedly disorganized hepatocyte arrangement (yellow arrows), cytoplasmic vacuolization (red arrows), and inflammatory cell infiltration (green arrows). In the PS-MP + SeNP group, the histopathological results showed significant improvement compared to the PS-MP group. The cytoplasmic vacuolation was relatively attenuated, although there was still evidence of inflammatory cell infiltration. The SeNP group did not differ significantly from the control group. Liver sections exhibited normal hepatocytes with intact cytoplasm, as well as intact nuclei, nucleoli, and central veins.

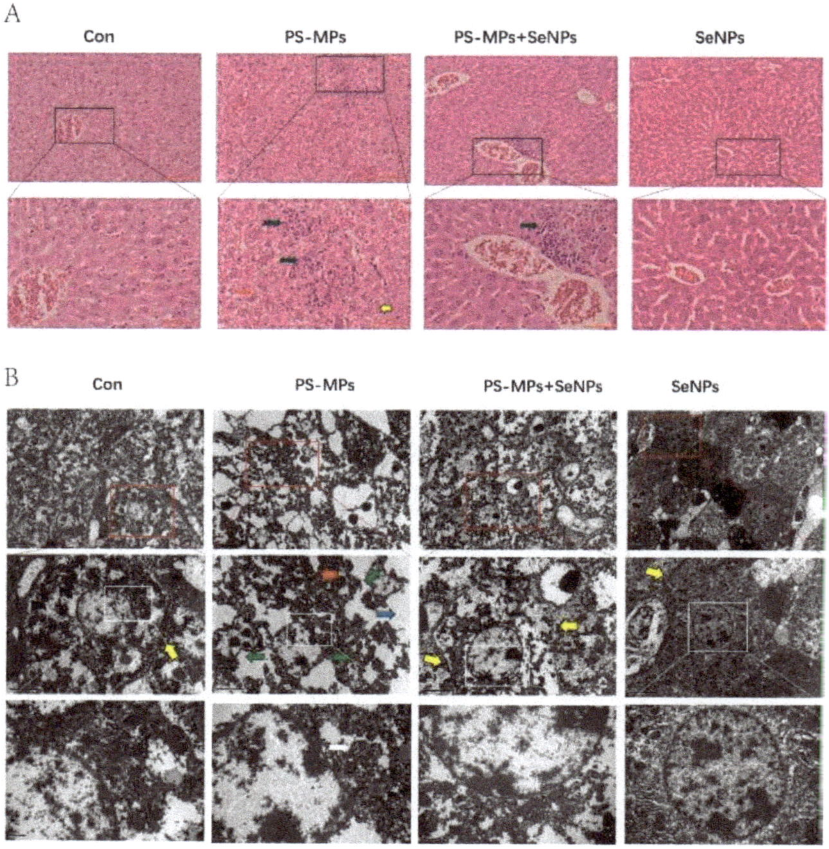

Figure 5. H&E stain images and electron microscopic images of liver tissue sections. (**A**) H&E stain map of mouse liver tissue. The overall magnification is 200× while the magnification of the black boxed section is 400×. Green arrows, inflammatory cell infiltration; yellow arrows, cytoplasmic vacuolation. (**B**) Transmission electron micrographs of mouse liver tissue. Red arrows: blurred cell membrane boundaries; yellow arrows: clear cell membrane boundaries; green arrows: distorted nuclei; white arrows: slightly abnormal mitochondrial structure with loosely arranged cristae; blue arrows: cytoplasmic vacuolation.

TEM was used to observe the cellular ultrastructure in liver tissue 28 days after molding, as shown in Figure 5B. After being exposed to PS-MPs, hepatocytes displayed distorted nuclei (indicated by green arrows), blurred cell membrane boundaries (indicated by red arrows), and cytoplasm filled with vacuoles (indicated by blue arrows) when observed at a magnification of 5000×. At 15,000× magnification, PS-MP exposure showed a slightly abnormal mitochondrial structure with loosely arranged cristae (white arrows). The histopathological findings in the PS-MP + SeNP group, on the other hand, were significantly improved, with no deformation of the nucleus and clear cell membrane boundaries. Cell membrane boundaries were clearer in the control, SeNP and PS-MP + SeNP groups (yellow arrows). The SeNP group did not show any notable distinction when compared to the control group. The findings from all these experiments clearly demonstrated that SeNPs exert a notable counteractive impact on liver damage caused by PS-MPs.

4.3.4. SeNPs Attenuates PS-MP-Induced Liver Function Impairment

In order to validate the protective effect of nano-selenium against liver injury caused by PS-MPs, we examined serum liver enzymes, such as aspartate transaminase (AST), alkaline phosphatase (ALP), and alanine aminotransferase (ALT), in accordance with histological findings. Levels of these enzymes indicative of liver injury were significantly elevated in the PS-MP group (10 mg/mL) compared to the normal group ($p < 0.01$). However, the increase was inhibited by SeNPs ($p < 0.01$) (Figure 6A–C). Furthermore, there was a notable rise in the fat content within the mouse tissues in the PS-MP group compared to the control group ($p < 0.01$). However, the PS-MP + SeNP group effectively mitigated the fat content increase caused by PS-MPs within the mouse tissues ($p < 0.01$) (Figure 6H).

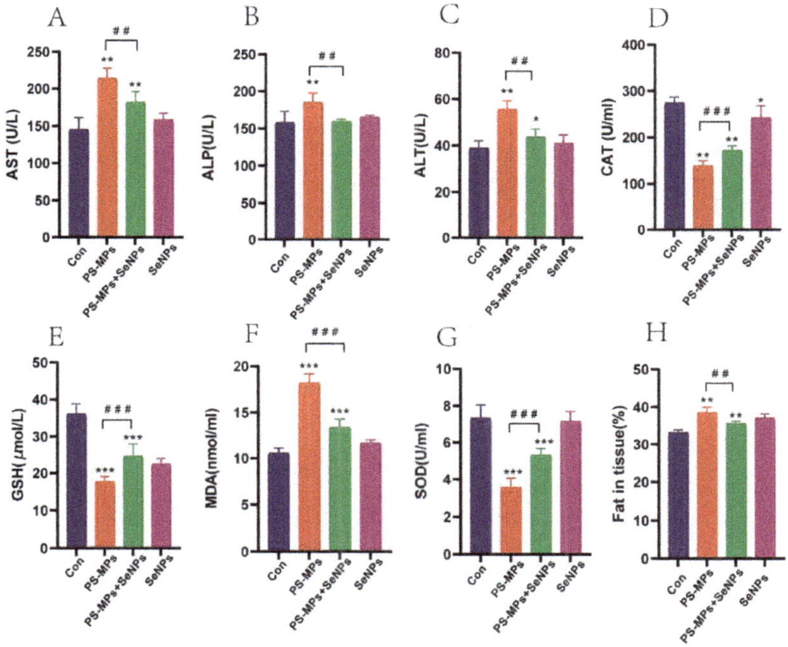

Figure 6. SeNPs attenuate PS-MP-induced liver function impairment. (**A**) Serum aspartate transaminase (AST) (**B**) serum alkaline phosphatase (ALP), (**C**) serum alanine aminotransferase (ALT), (**D**) catalase (CAT), (**E**) glutathione (GSH) (**F**) malondialdehyde (MDA), (**G**) superoxide dismutase (SOD), (**H**) fat content in tissues. The data are presented as the average plus or minus the standard deviation (n = 6). *: $p < 0.05$, **: $p < 0.01$, ***: $p < 0.001$. p-values of groups compared with each other: ##: $p < 0.01$, ###: $p < 0.001$.

4.3.5. Protective Impact of Nano-Selenium on Oxidative Stress Caused by PS-MPs

The MDA content was significantly increased in the PS-MP-exposed group compared to the control group, while the elevated MDA content caused by PS-MPs was significantly reduced in the PS-MP + SeNP group (Figure 6F). In contrast, CAT ($p < 0.01$), GSH ($p < 0.001$), and SOD ($p < 0.001$) activities were significantly decreased in the PS-MP group compared to the control group. In contrast, the PS-MP + SeNP group significantly elevated the decrease in CAT, GSH, and SOD activities caused by PS-MPs (Figure 6D,E,G). These results suggest that PS-MP exposure led to an imbalance of the redox system in mouse liver tissues, resulting in oxidative damage.

4.3.6. Effect of SeNPs on PS-MP-Induced Liver-Injury-Related Proteins Through Regulation of the NF-κB/NLRP3 Inflammatory Pathway

NF-κB in the PS-MP group was mainly expressed in the central vein, while NLRP3 was mainly expressed in the cells surrounding the central vein (Figure 7A) The protein expression levels of NF-κB, P-NF-κB, TNF-α, Cleaved Caspase1, Caspase1, NLRP3, and IL-1β were significantly higher in the PS-MP group than in the control group ($p < 0.01$). The protein expression levels were all significantly lower in the PS-MP + SeNP group compared to the PS-MP group ($p < 0.01$) (Figure 7B,C). These results suggest that SeNPs attenuated the liver inflammatory injury induced by PS-MPs by regulating the NF-κB/NLRP3 inflammasome pathway.

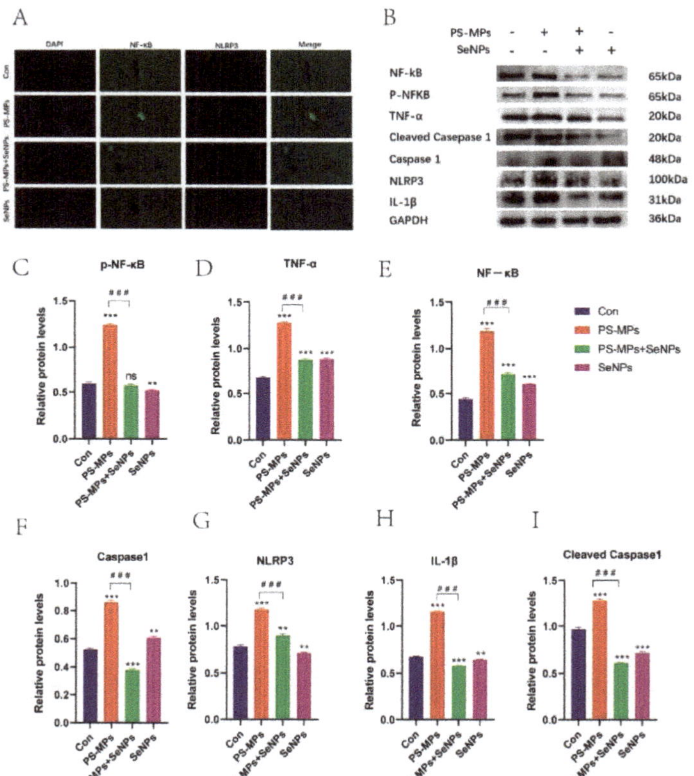

Figure 7. Effects of SeNPs on PS-MP-induced liver-injury-related proteins by modulating the NF-κB/NLRP3 inflammatory vesicle pathway. (**A**) Immunofluorescence expression of NF-κB protein and NLRP3 protein in the liver of each group of mice. (**B**) Protein blots of NF-κB, P-NF-κB, TNF-α, Cleaved Caspase1, Caspase1, NLRP3, IL-1β (n = 3). (**C**–**I**) Quantitative expression of these proteins (n = 3). **: $p < 0.01$, ***: $p < 0.001$, ns: not statistically significant. p-values of groups compared with each other: ###: $p < 0.001$.

4.3.7. Effects of SeNPs on Genes Related to PS-MP-Induced Liver Injury Through Regulation of the NF-κB/NLRP3 Inflammatory Vesicle Pathway

The gene expression levels of NF-κB, TNF-α, Caspase1, NLRP3, and IL-1β were significantly higher in the PS-MP group than in the control group ($p < 0.01$). The gene expression levels were all significantly lower in the PS-MP + SeNP group compared to the PS-MP group ($p < 0.01$) (Figure 8A–E). These results suggest that nano-sized selenium was able to attenuate the inflammatory liver injury induced by PS-MPs.

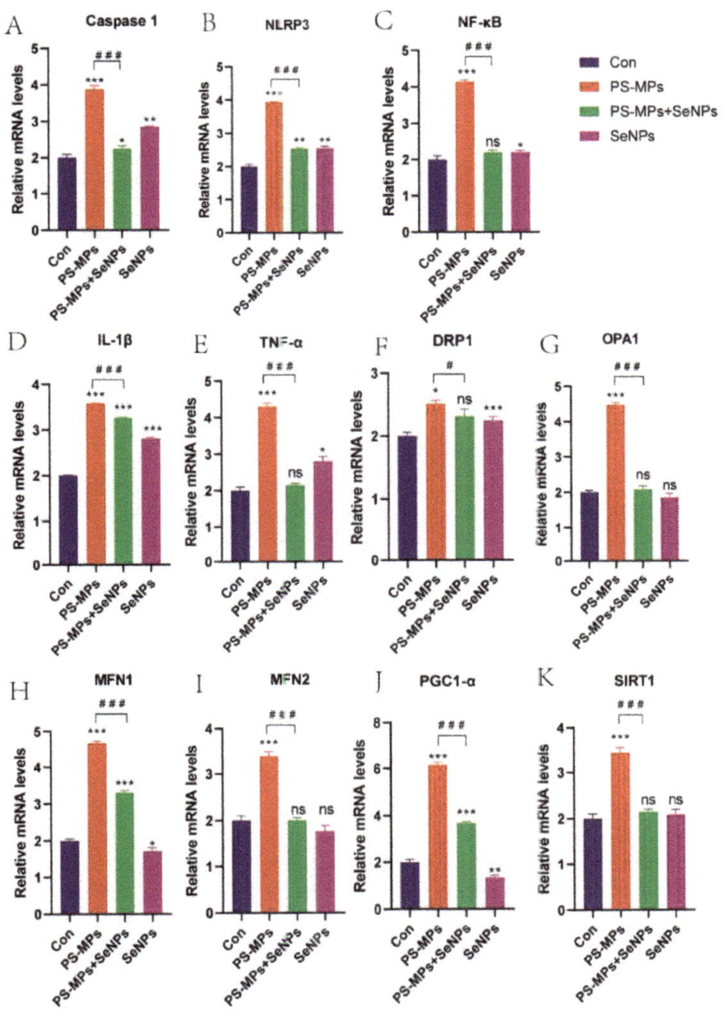

Figure 8. Measurement using quantitative real-time fluorescence qPCR. (**A–E**) Levels of gene expression related to inflammation. (**F–K**) Levels of gene expression linked to mitochondria. *: $p < 0.05$, **: $p < 0.01$, ***: $p < 0.001$, ns: not statistically significant. p-values of groups compared with each other: #: $p < 0.05$, ###: $p < 0.001$. ns: not statistically significant.

4.3.8. SeNPs Attenuate PS-MP-Induced Mitochondrial Dysfunction

Compared with the control group, the mRNA levels of mitochondria-related genes, such as OPA1, DRP1, MFN1, and MFN2, were significantly higher in the PS-MP group. (Figure 8F–K), indicating accelerated mitochondrial division and fusion. Among them, MFN1 is involved in the attachment of nearby mitochondria, maintenance of mitochondrial membrane potential, and apoptosis. MFN2 is a multifunctional protein located in the outer mitochondrial membrane, controlling mitochondrial fusion and physical interactions with other organelles. However, after co-treatment with SeNPs, the mRNA levels of all of them were significantly down-regulated. Furthermore, taken together, these results suggest that SeNPs have a protective effect on mitochondria.

5. Discussion

Accumulation of microplastics causes oxidative stress, inflammation, and apoptosis-related toxic effects in the liver, as well as disturbances in glucose and lipid metabolism in the liver [33]. The liver plays a crucial role in the storage, conversion, and breakdown of medications [34]. Several studies have been conducted on the mammalian biosafety of PS-MPs [35]. However, studies on the protective effects and molecular mechanisms of combined SeNPs against PS-MP-induced liver injury have not been reported. This study has confirmed for the first time that SeNPs reduce liver damage caused by microplastics by regulating inflammation mediated by the NF-κB/NLRP3 inflammatory pathway. This study confirmed that nano-selenium effectively reduced liver damage induced by PS-MPs, as observed through histopathological examination and serum biochemical analysis. Additionally, it unveiled the precise molecular mechanisms of nano-selenium in terms of mitochondrial dynamics, oxidative stress, and inflammation.

First, we determined in vitro experiments with normal mouse NCTC1469 hepatocytes that PS-MPs have a damaging effect on hepatocytes, while SeNPs have a proliferative effect on hepatocytes. The mitochondria primarily metabolize oxygen in aerobic organisms. Reactive oxygen species (ROS) are typically generated by organisms during cellular respiration. They are primarily found in liver cells and immune cells, where they promote cellular maturation and programmed cell death [36,37]. Excessive generation of ROS can result from different cellular stresses, and prolonged exposure to elevated levels of ROS is a significant factor contributing to numerous pathological conditions [38–41]. The findings of this study align with previous research on the harmful effects of microplastics on various tissues. This indicates that the inflammation caused by microplastics is strongly linked to the excessive buildup of ROS, which triggers inflammatory signaling and leads to inflammatory damage [42]. On the other hand, selenium (Se) acts as a strong catalyst for glutathione peroxidase (GPx) [43]. GPx, an important selenoprotein within the body, plays a crucial role in regulating the excessive generation of radicals in areas of inflammation. It also ensures the maintenance of the intracellular redox equilibrium and provides antioxidant properties to safeguard healthy cells against oxidative harm caused by ROS. Furthermore, studies have demonstrated that the augmentation of Se-GPx activity in the livers of mice leads to an improved capacity of the antioxidant system to safeguard against harm [44]. The balance between oxidants and antioxidants is controlled by the activity of Se-GPx [45]. Nano-selenium has strong hepatoprotective bioactivities and may be an antioxidant treatment [46]. Moderate amounts of nano-selenium in vivo are effective in ameliorating liver injury induced by PS-MPs. Therefore, nano-selenium supplementation can attenuate oxidative stress (ROS) induced by PS-MP exposure.

To summarize, our experiments conducted in a controlled environment demonstrated that PS-MPs increase the levels of reactive oxygen within cells, while the inclusion of SeNPs mitigated the harm inflicted on liver cells by PS-MPs. Based on this foundation, we performed in vivo tests on ICR mice using varying doses of PS-MPs. A previous study showed that polystyrene microplastics induced the formation of extracellular traps in macrophages, activating the ROS/TGF-β/Smad2/3 signaling axis, leading to an inflammatory response and epithelial–mesenchymal transition in hepatocytes [47]. The impairment of hepatocytes can result in the secretion of diverse enzymes and a prompt corresponding response, indicating significant liver damage [48]. In this experiment, several biochemical indices related to mouse liver were evaluated by oral administration of PS-MPs. These indicators play a crucial role in the metabolism of mammalian liver cells. The results of the test showed that there were significant differences in the indicators related to liver damage as the concentration of PS-MPs increased and that there was accumulative effect of concentration. The results showed that exposure to different concentrations of PS-MPs caused an increase in various biochemical parameters of liver function in mice, as well as an increase in tissue, fat content, and liver coefficients, indicating that liver cells were damaged.

Therefore, among the animal tests with different PS-MP concentrations, we chose the concentration of PS-MPs with the most significant liver damage (10 mg/kg/d) for a further

test to explore the combination with SeNPs. The results showed that the levels of several antioxidant enzymes in the serum of mice were significantly decreased after exposure to PS-MPs, while the levels of MDA increased significantly. Among them, GSH plays an important role in scavenging reactive oxygen species, SOD plays a role in scavenging free radicals, and CAT plays a role in scavenging hydrogen peroxide in the body [49]. MDA is a product of lipid peroxidation, which can be used as an indicator of oxidative damage [50]. These results suggest that exposure to PS-MPs decreases the level of antioxidant defenses in mice, leading to increased oxidative stress. However, the impairment of hepatic oxidative stress by PS-MPs was significantly reversed by the addition of SeNPs.

Meanwhile, a study showed that exposure to PS-MPs induced apoptosis and pyroptosis in granulosa cells in rat ovaries, leading to an increase in inflammatory markers, and the mechanism of action was associated with activation of the NLRP3/Caspase1 pathway [51]. A study of microplastics in brain injury also confirmed that microplastics disrupt mitochondrial function and activate AMPK signaling, leading to inflammation in the brain. This evidence suggests that microplastics damage tissues through different mechanisms and that elevated inflammatory markers in the liver are a sign of the damage they cause [52–54]. Aberrant expression of NF-κB pathway pro-inflammatory cytokines is a major feature of the inflammatory response [55–57].

The findings indicated that PS-MPs activate the NF-κB pathway in the mouse liver, functioning as a pivotal hub for signaling, an emergency sensor, and being responsive to nearly all hazardous cues [58]. Moreover, it was evident that PS-MPs stimulate NLRP3 inflammatory vesicles within the liver. NLRP3, one of the NOD-like receptors, stands out as the most adaptable and medically important inflammatory vesicle, triggered by a diverse range of stimuli that are not commonly seen [59]. Increased mitochondrial cleavage has been reported to activate the generation of NLRP3 inflammatory vesicles [60,61]. In addition, NF-κB promotes the synthesis of mRNAs for several inflammation-related genes, including NLRP3 [62,63]. The findings indicate that PS-MPs have the ability to trigger inflammation in NLRP3 vesicles, leading to scorch-induced cell death. In addition, activation of the NF-κB pathway may be one of the mechanisms of NLRP3 inflammatory vesicle initiation. Activation of NLRP3 inflammatory vesicles initiates the NF-κB pathway and mediates cleavage. NLRP3 inflammatory vesicles can be activated by inflammatory factors, mitochondrial reactive oxygen species, and lysosomal enzyme damage [64–66]. The NF-κB pathway [67] can be activated by oxidative stress, resulting in the release of inflammatory factors and ultimately leading to the occurrence of NLRP3 inflammatory-vesicle-induced scorch death. Thus, our hypothesis is that the NF-κB signaling pathway could be activated and NLRP3 inflammatory-vesicle-induced scorch death could be mediated by PS-MP-induced oxidative stress. Although the precise mechanism is still unknown, this offers a solid foundation for conducting exposure studies on PS-MPs.

Mitochondria play a role in multiple crucial cellular functions, and excessive exposure to PS-MPs disrupts the dynamics of mitochondria, ultimately resulting in the death of liver cells in mice. SIRT1 positively regulates pGC1-α, a crucial mediator of mitochondrial biogenesis, as well as the fusion and fission processes of mitochondria [68]. The findings of this test indicate that PS-MPs lead to increased mitochondrial fragmentation, decreased merging and formation, and ultimately oxidative stress and apoptosis by enhancing mRNA expression of multiple genes associated with mitochondria [69,70]. SeNPs have been found to improve the function of the mitochondrial electron transport chain and control the production of new mitochondria [71,72]. The findings indicate that SeNPs have the ability to preserve the balance of mitochondrial dynamics by controlling the proteins responsible for both mitochondrial division and merging.

It is important to take into account various restrictions in our research. For instance, our attempts to delve deeper into the involvement of oxidative stress in the activation of NLRP3 inflammatory vesicles were unsuccessful. In our present investigation, we solely investigated the mechanisms linked to NF-κB/NLRP3 induction in liver cells due to exposure to PS-MPs, without analyzing the correlation between alternative programmed cellular pathways and diverse forms of cell death. Our future studies will center around these areas.

6. Conclusions

The current research illustrates that PS-MPs exhibit cumulative impacts at varying levels of exposure. Oral administration of PS-MPs resulted in the activation of the NF-κB/NLRP3 inflammatory signaling pathway in the liver of mice, resulting in a certain degree of liver damage. Mitochondrial pathway activation caused oxidative stress, inflammation, and hepatocyte scorching, resulting in hepatocyte damage, liver dysfunction, and hepatotoxicity. On the other hand, the inclusion of SeNPs greatly reduces the liver damage caused by microplastics. Nano-selenium, a trace element, is crucial in the pathophysiological mechanisms of organisms. The data and references presented in this study can be used to evaluate the biological hazard of orally consuming environmentally exposed PS-MPs in mice. The findings of the research could additionally aid in the advancement of policies aimed at preventing and managing plastic pollution.

Author Contributions: Y.L.: Writing—original draft, Conceptualization, Methodology, Data curation. Q.S.: Software, Validation, Writing—review and editing, Formal analysis. D.Z.: Data curation, Supervision, Project administration, Funding acquisition. J.L.: Data curation, Supervision, Project administration, Funding acquisition. All authors have read and agreed to the published version of the manuscript.

Funding: This research received no external funding.

Institutional Review Board Statement: The study was conducted in accordance with the Declaration of Helsinki and approved by the Institutional Review Board of Animal Experimental Ethical Inspection of Laboratory Animal Centre, Huazhong Agriculture University (SYXK2020-0084, 11 July 2023).

Informed Consent Statement: Not applicable.

Data Availability Statement: The original contributions presented in the study are included in the article, further inquiries can be directed to the corresponding author.

Conflicts of Interest: The authors declare that they have no known competing financial interests or personal relationships that could have appeared to influence the work reported in this paper.

References

1. Amélineau, F.; Bonnet, D.; Heitz, O.; Mortreux, V.; Harding, A.M.A.; Karnovsky, N.; Walkusz, W.; Fort, J.; Grémillet, D. Microplastic pollution in the Greenland Sea: Background levels and selective contamination of planktivorous diving seabirds. *Environ. Pollut.* **2016**, *219*, 1131–1139. [CrossRef] [PubMed]
2. Chae, Y.; An, Y.J. Effects of micro- and nanoplastics on aquatic ecosystems: Current research trends and perspectives. *Mar. Pollut. Bull.* **2017**, *124*, 624–632. [CrossRef] [PubMed]
3. Peeken, I.; Primpke, S.; Beyer, B.; Gütermann, J.; Katlein, C.; Krumpen, T.; Bergmann, M.; Hehemann, L.; Gerdts, G. Arctic sea ice is an important temporal sink and means of transport for microplastic. *Nat. Commun.* **2018**, *9*, 1505. [CrossRef] [PubMed]
4. Lambert, S.; Wagner, M. Exploring the effects of microplastics in freshwater environments. *Integr. Environ. Assess. Manag.* **2016**, *12*, 404–405. [CrossRef] [PubMed]
5. Law, K.L.; Thompson, R.C. Oceans. Microplastics in the seas. *Science* **2014**, *345*, 144–145. [CrossRef]
6. Bouwmeester, H.; Hollman, P.C.; Peters, R.J. Potential Health Impact of Environmentally Released Micro- and Nanoplastics in the Human Food Production Chain: Experiences from Nanotoxicology. *Environ. Sci. Technol.* **2015**, *49*, 8932–8947. [CrossRef]
7. Cózar, A.; Echevarría, F.; González-Gordillo, J.I.; Irigoien, X.; Úbeda, B.; Hernández-León, S.; Palma, Á.T.; Navarro, S.; García-de-Lomas, J.; Ruiz, A.; et al. Plastic debris in the open ocean. *Proc. Natl. Acad. Sci. USA* **2014**, *111*, 10239–10244. [CrossRef]
8. Sharma, S.; Chatterjee, S. Microplastic pollution, a threat to marine ecosystem and human health: A short review. *Environ. Sci. Pollut. Res. Int.* **2017**, *24*, 21530–21547. [CrossRef]
9. Yang, X.; Man, Y.B.; Wong, M.H.; Owen, R.B.; Chow, K.L. Environmental health impacts of microplastics exposure on structural organization levels in the human body. *Sci. Total Environ.* **2022**, *825*, 154025. [CrossRef]
10. Cox, K.D.; Covernton, G.A.; Davies, H.L.; Dower, J.F.; Juanes, F.; Dudas, S.E. Human Consumption of Microplastics. *Environ. Sci. Technol.* **2019**, *53*, 7068–7074. [CrossRef]
11. Fan, X.; Wei, X.; Hu, H.; Zhang, B.; Yang, D.; Du, H.; Zhu, R.; Sun, X.; Oh, Y.; Gu, N. Effects of oral administration of polystyrene nanoplastics on plasma glucose metabolism in mice. *Chemosphere* **2022**, *288*, 132607. [CrossRef] [PubMed]

12. Liang, B.; Zhong, Y.; Huang, Y.; Lin, X.; Liu, J.; Lin, L.; Hu, M.; Jiang, J.; Dai, M.; Wang, B.; et al. Underestimated health risks: Polystyrene micro- and nanoplastics jointly induce intestinal barrier dysfunction by ROS-mediated epithelial cell apoptosis. *Part. Fibre Toxicol.* **2021**, *18*, 20. [CrossRef] [PubMed]
13. Meng, X.; Zhang, J.; Wang, W.; Gonzalez-Gil, G.; Vrouwenvelder, J.S.; Li, Z. Effects of nano- and microplastics on kidney: Physicochemical properties, bioaccumulation, oxidative stress and immunoreaction. *Chemosphere* **2022**, *288*, 132631. [CrossRef] [PubMed]
14. Sun, M.; Ding, R.; Ma, Y.; Sun, Q.; Ren, X.; Sun, Z.; Duan, J. Cardiovascular toxicity assessment of polyethylene nanoplastics on developing zebrafish embryos. *Chemosphere* **2021**, *282*, 131124. [CrossRef]
15. Deng, Y.; Zhang, Y.; Lemos, B.; Ren, H. Tissue accumulation of microplastics in mice and biomarker responses suggest widespread health risks of exposure. *Sci. Rep.* **2017**, *7*, 46687. [CrossRef]
16. Shin, H.S.; Lee, S.H.; Moon, H.J.; So, Y.H.; Lee, H.R.; Lee, E.H.; Jung, E.M. Exposure to polystyrene particles causes anxiety-, depression-like behavior and abnormal social behavior in mice. *J. Hazard. Mater.* **2023**, *454*, 131465. [CrossRef]
17. Yang, Y.F.; Chen, C.Y.; Lu, T.H.; Liao, C.M. Toxicity-based toxicokinetic/toxicodynamic assessment for bioaccumulation of polystyrene microplastics in mice. *J. Hazard. Mater.* **2019**, *366*, 703–713. [CrossRef]
18. Núñez, M.; Soriano, V. Hepatotoxicity of antiretrovirals: Incidence, mechanisms and management. *Drug Saf.* **2005**, *28*, 53–66. [CrossRef]
19. Powell, E.E.; Wong, V.W.; Rinella, M. Non-alcoholic fatty liver disease. *Lancet* **2021**, *397*, 2212–2224. [CrossRef]
20. Lu, L.; Wan, Z.; Luo, T.; Fu, Z.; Jin, Y. Polystyrene microplastics induce gut microbiota dysbiosis and hepatic lipid metabolism disorder in mice. *Sci. Total Environ.* **2018**, *631–632*, 449–458. [CrossRef]
21. Cheng, H.; Duan, Z.; Wu, Y.; Wang, Y.; Zhang, H.; Shi, Y.; Zhang, H.; Wei, Y.; Sun, H. Immunotoxicity responses to polystyrene nanoplastics and their related mechanisms in the liver of zebrafish (*Danio rerio*) larvae. *Environ. Int.* **2022**, *161*, 107128. [CrossRef] [PubMed]
22. Huang, T.; Zhang, W.; Lin, T.; Liu, S.; Sun, Z.; Liu, F.; Yuan, Y.; Xiang, X.; Kuang, H.; Yang, B.; et al. Maternal exposure to polystyrene nanoplastics during gestation and lactation induces hepatic and testicular toxicity in male mouse offspring. *Food Chem. Toxicol.* **2022**, *160*, 112803. [CrossRef] [PubMed]
23. Kieliszek, M. Selenium-Fascinating Microelement, Properties and Sources in Food. *Molecules* **2019**, *24*, 1298. [CrossRef] [PubMed]
24. Kieliszek, M.; Błażejak, S. Selenium: Significance, and outlook for supplementation. *Nutrition* **2013**, *29*, 713–718. [CrossRef]
25. Yang, J.; Yang, H. Recent development in Se-enriched yeast, lactic acid bacteria and bifidobacteria. *Crit. Rev. Food Sci. Nutr.* **2023**, *63*, 411–425. [CrossRef]
26. Kato, T.; Read, R.; Rozga, J.; Burk, R.F. Evidence for intestinal release of absorbed selenium in a form with high hepatic extraction. *Am. J. Physiol.* **1992**, *262*, G854–G858. [CrossRef]
27. Luo, J.; Li, X.; Li, X.; He, Y.; Zhang, M.; Cao, C.; Wang, K. Selenium-Rich Yeast protects against aluminum-induced peroxidation of lipide and inflammation in mouse liver. *Biometals* **2018**, *31*, 1051–1059. [CrossRef]
28. Reja, M.; Makar, M.; Visaria, A.; Marino, D.; Rustgi, V. Increased serum selenium levels are associated with reduced risk of advanced liver fibrosis and all-cause mortality in NAFLD patients: National Health and Nutrition Examination Survey (NHANES) III. *Ann. Hepatol.* **2020**, *19*, 635–640. [CrossRef]
29. Zhang, X.; Xia, H.; Wang, J.; Leng, R.; Zhou, X.; Gao, Q.; He, K.; Liu, D.; Huang, B. Effect of selenium-enriched kiwifruit on body fat reduction and liver protection in hyperlipidaemic mice. *Food Funct.* **2021**, *12*, 2044–2057. [CrossRef]
30. Ge, J.; Guo, K.; Zhang, C.; Talukder, M.; Lv, M.W.; Li, J.Y.; Li, J.L. Comparison of nanoparticle-selenium, selenium-enriched yeast and sodium selenite on the alleviation of cadmium-induced inflammation via NF-kB/IκB pathway in heart. *Sci. Total Environ.* **2021**, *773*, 145442. [CrossRef]
31. Wang, H.; Zhang, J.; Yu, H. Elemental selenium at nano size possesses lower toxicity without compromising the fundamental effect on selenoenzymes: Comparison with selenomethionine in mice. *Free Radic. Biol. Med.* **2007**, *42*, 1524–1533. [CrossRef] [PubMed]
32. Zhang, H.; Li, Z.; Dai, C.; Wang, P.; Fan, S.; Yu, B.; Qu, Y. Antibacterial properties and mechanism of selenium nanoparticles synthesized by *Providencia* sp. DCX. *Environ. Res.* **2021**, *194*, 110630. [CrossRef] [PubMed]
33. Mu, Y.; Sun, J.; Li, Z.; Zhang, W.; Liu, Z.; Li, C.; Peng, C.; Cui, G.; Shao, H.; Du, Z. Activation of pyroptosis and ferroptosis is involved in the hepatotoxicity induced by polystyrene microplastics in mice. *Chemosphere* **2022**, *291*, 132944. [CrossRef] [PubMed]
34. Liu, P.; Li, H.; Li, R.; Geng, Y.; Gong, J.; Xu, H.; Xu, Z.; Shi, J. Nanoencapsulation of chitooligosaccharides enhances its oral bioavailability and anti-liver fibrotic effects. *Food Res. Int.* **2022**, *157*, 111471. [CrossRef] [PubMed]
35. Jia, R.; Han, J.; Liu, X.; Li, K.; Lai, W.; Bian, L.; Yan, J.; Xi, Z. Exposure to Polypropylene Microplastics via Oral Ingestion Induces Colonic Apoptosis and Intestinal Barrier Damage through Oxidative Stress and Inflammation in Mice. *Toxics* **2023**, *11*, 127. [CrossRef]
36. Jakubczyk, K.; Dec, K.; Kałduńska, J.; Kawczuga, D.; Kochman, J.; Janda, K. Reactive oxygen species—Sources, functions, oxidative damage. *Pol. Merkur. Lek.* **2020**, *48*, 124–127.
37. Zhou, Z.; Ni, K.; Deng, H.; Chen, X. Dancing with reactive oxygen species generation and elimination in nanotheranostics for disease treatment. *Adv. Drug Deliv. Rev.* **2020**, *158*, 73–90. [CrossRef]
38. Boveris, A.; Chance, B. The mitochondrial generation of hydrogen peroxide. General properties and effect of hyperbaric oxygen. *Biochem. J.* **1973**, *134*, 707–716. [CrossRef]

39. Brieger, K.; Schiavone, S.; Miller, F.J., Jr.; Krause, K.H. Reactive oxygen species: From health to disease. *Swiss Med. Wkly.* **2012**, *142*, w13659. [CrossRef]
40. Klaunig, J.E. Oxidative Stress and Cancer. *Curr. Pharm. Des.* **2018**, *24*, 4771–4778. [CrossRef]
41. Liochev, S.I. Reactive oxygen species and the free radical theory of aging. *Free Radic. Biol. Med.* **2013**, *60*, 1–4. [CrossRef]
42. Li, X.; Bai, R.; Bai, Y.; Shi, X.; Yang, Y.; Xu, S. ROS-mediated PPAR/RXR inhibition contributes to acetochlor-induced apoptosis and autophagy in Ctenopharyngodon idella hepatic cells. *Fish. Shellfish Immunol.* **2022**, *128*, 684–694. [CrossRef] [PubMed]
43. Shen, Y.; Huang, H.; Wang, Y.; Yang, R.; Ke, X. Antioxidant effects of Se-glutathione peroxidase in alcoholic liver disease. *J. Trace Elem. Med. Biol.* **2022**, *74*, 127048. [CrossRef] [PubMed]
44. Duntas, L.H. Selenium and inflammation: Underlying anti-inflammatory mechanisms. *Horm. Metab. Res.* **2009**, *41*, 443–447. [CrossRef] [PubMed]
45. Chatziargyriou, V.; Dailianis, S. The role of selenium-dependent glutathione peroxidase (Se-GPx) against oxidative and genotoxic effects of mercury in haemocytes of mussel *Mytilus galloprovincialis* (Lmk.). *Toxicol. In Vitro* **2010**, *24*, 1363–1372. [CrossRef] [PubMed]
46. Rua, R.M.; Ojeda, M.L.; Nogales, F.; Rubio, J.M.; Romero-Gómez, M.; Funuyet, J.; Murillo, M.L.; Carreras, O. Serum selenium levels and oxidative balance as differential markers in hepatic damage caused by alcohol. *Life Sci.* **2014**, *94*, 158–163. [CrossRef]
47. Wang, S.; Chen, L.; Shi, X.; Wang, Y.; Xu, S. Polystyrene microplastics-induced macrophage extracellular traps contributes to liver fibrotic injury by activating ROS/TGF-β/Smad2/3 signaling axis. *Environ. Pollut.* **2023**, *324*, 121388. [CrossRef]
48. Qin, X.; Wang, X.; Tian, M.; Dong, Z.; Wang, J.; Wang, C.; Huang, Q. The role of Andrographolide in the prevention and treatment of liver diseases. *Phytomedicine* **2023**, *109*, 154537. [CrossRef]
49. Yun, S.H.; Moon, Y.S.; Sohn, S.H.; Jang, I.S. Effects of cyclic heat stress or vitamin C supplementation during cyclic heat stress on HSP70, inflammatory cytokines, and the antioxidant defense system in Sprague Dawley rats. *Exp. Anim.* **2012**, *61*, 543–553. [CrossRef]
50. Impellizzeri, D.; Cordaro, M.; Campolo, M.; Gugliandolo, E.; Esposito, E.; Benedetto, F.; Cuzzocrea, S.; Navarra, M. Anti-inflammatory and Antioxidant Effects of Flavonoid-Rich Fraction of Bergamot Juice (BJe) in a Mice Model of Intestinal Ischemia/Reperfusion Injury. *Front. Pharmacol.* **2016**, *7*, 203. [CrossRef]
51. Wang, P.X.; Zhang, X.J.; Luo, P.; Jiang, X.; Zhang, P.; Guo, J.; Zhao, G.N.; Zhu, X.; Zhang, Y.; Yang, S.; et al. Hepatocyte TRAF3 promotes liver steatosis and systemic insulin resistance through targeting TAK1-dependent signalling. *Nat. Commun.* **2016**, *7*, 10592. [CrossRef] [PubMed]
52. Hou, J.; Lei, Z.; Cui, L.; Hou, Y.; Yang, L.; An, R.; Wang, Q.; Li, S.; Zhang, H.; Zhang, L. Polystyrene microplastics lead to pyroptosis and apoptosis of ovarian granulosa cells via NLRP3/Caspase-1 signaling pathway in rats. *Ecotoxicol. Environ. Saf.* **2021**, *212*, 112012. [CrossRef] [PubMed]
53. Hu, M.; Palić, D. Micro- and nano-plastics activation of oxidative and inflammatory adverse outcome pathways. *Redox Biol.* **2020**, *37*, 101620. [CrossRef] [PubMed]
54. Yin, K.; Lu, H.; Zhang, Y.; Hou, L.; Meng, X.; Li, J.; Zhao, H.; Xing, M. Secondary brain injury after polystyrene microplastic-induced intracerebral hemorrhage is associated with inflammation and pyroptosis. *Chem. Biol. Interact.* **2022**, *367*, 110180. [CrossRef] [PubMed]
55. Cao, H.; Gao, F.; Xia, B.; Xiao, Q.; Guo, X.; Hu, G.; Zhang, C. The co-induced effects of molybdenum and cadmium on the mRNA expression of inflammatory cytokines and trace element contents in duck kidneys. *Ecotoxicol. Environ. Saf.* **2016**, *133*, 157–163. [CrossRef]
56. He, F.; Huang, Y.; Song, Z.; Zhou, H.J.; Zhang, H.; Perry, R.J.; Shulman, G.I.; Min, W. Mitophagy-mediated adipose inflammation contributes to type 2 diabetes with hepatic insulin resistance. *J. Exp. Med.* **2021**, *218*. [CrossRef]
57. Yang, Z.; Wang, S.; Liu, H.; Xu, S. MAPK/iNOS pathway is involved in swine kidney necrosis caused by cadmium exposure. *Environ. Pollut.* **2021**, *274*, 116497. [CrossRef]
58. Kracht, M.; Müller-Ladner, U.; Schmitz, M.L. Mutual regulation of metabolic processes and proinflammatory NF-κB signaling. *J. Allergy Clin. Immunol.* **2020**, *146*, 694–705. [CrossRef]
59. Baroja-Mazo, A.; Martín-Sánchez, F.; Gomez, A.I.; Martínez, C.M.; Amores-Iniesta, J.; Compan, V.; Barberà-Cremades, M.; Yagüe, J.; Ruiz-Ortiz, E.; Antón, J.; et al. The NLRP3 inflammasome is released as a particulate danger signal that amplifies the inflammatory response. *Nat. Immunol.* **2014**, *15*, 738–748. [CrossRef]
60. Angajala, A.; Lim, S.; Phillips, J.B.; Kim, J.H.; Yates, C.; You, Z.; Tan, M. Diverse Roles of Mitochondria in Immune Responses: Novel Insights into Immuno-Metabolism. *Front. Immunol.* **2018**, *9*, 1605. [CrossRef]
61. Mangan, M.S.J.; Olhava, E.J.; Roush, W.R.; Seidel, H.M.; Glick, G.D.; Latz, E. Targeting the NLRP3 inflammasome in inflammatory diseases. *Nat. Rev. Drug Discov.* **2018**, *17*, 588–606. [CrossRef] [PubMed]
62. An, Y.; Zhang, H.; Wang, C.; Jiao, F.; Xu, H.; Wang, X.; Luan, W.; Ma, F.; Ni, L.; Tang, X.; et al. Activation of ROS/MAPKs/NF-κB/NLRP3 and inhibition of efferocytosis in osteoclast-mediated diabetic osteoporosis. *FASEB J.* **2019**, *33*, 12515–12527. [CrossRef] [PubMed]
63. Park, E.; Chung, S.W. ROS-mediated autophagy increases intracellular iron levels and ferroptosis by ferritin and transferrin receptor regulation. *Cell Death Dis.* **2019**, *10*, 822. [CrossRef] [PubMed]
64. Dostert, C.; Pétrilli, V.; Van Bruggen, R.; Steele, C.; Mossman, B.T.; Tschopp, J. Innate immune activation through Nalp3 inflammasome sensing of asbestos and silica. *Science* **2008**, *320*, 674–677. [CrossRef] [PubMed]

65. Hornung, V.; Bauernfeind, F.; Halle, A.; Samstad, E.O.; Kono, H.; Rock, K.L.; Fitzgerald, K.A.; Latz, E. Silica crystals and aluminum salts activate the NALP3 inflammasome through phagosomal destabilization. *Nat. Immunol.* **2008**, *9*, 847–856. [CrossRef]
66. Pétrilli, V.; Papin, S.; Dostert, C.; Mayor, A.; Martinon, F.; Tschopp, J. Activation of the NALP3 inflammasome is triggered by low intracellular potassium concentration. *Cell Death Differ.* **2007**, *14*, 1583–1589. [CrossRef]
67. Purdy, M.; Kokki, M.; Anttila, M.; Aspinen, S.; Juvonen, P.; Selander, T.; Kokki, H.; Pulkki, K.; Eskelinen, M. Does Post-Surgery Placement of Rectus Sheath Block Analgesia Alter the Oxidative Stress Biomarker 8-OHdG Concentrations: A Randomised Trial of Patients with Cancer and Benign Disease. *Cancer Genom. Proteom.* **2016**, *13*, 239–244.
68. Nisr, R.B.; Shah, D.S.; Ganley, I.G.; Hundal, H.S. Proinflammatory NFkB signalling promotes mitochondrial dysfunction in skeletal muscle in response to cellular fuel overloading. *Cell Mol. Life Sci.* **2019**, *76*, 4887–4904. [CrossRef]
69. Li, C.X.; Gao, J.G.; Wan, X.Y.; Chen, Y.; Xu, C.F.; Feng, Z.M.; Zeng, H.; Lin, Y.M.; Ma, H.; Xu, P.; et al. Allyl isothiocyanate ameliorates lipid accumulation and inflammation in nonalcoholic fatty liver disease via the Sirt1/AMPK and NF-κB signaling pathways. *World J. Gastroenterol.* **2019**, *25*, 5120–5133. [CrossRef]
70. Li, S.; Baiyun, R.; Lv, Z.; Li, J.; Han, D.; Zhao, W.; Yu, L.; Deng, N.; Liu, Z.; Zhang, Z. Exploring the kidney hazard of exposure to mercuric chloride in mice: Disorder of mitochondrial dynamics induces oxidative stress and results in apoptosis. *Chemosphere* **2019**, *234*, 822–829. [CrossRef]
71. Arthur, J.R.; Nicol, F.; Beckett, G.J. The role of selenium in thyroid hormone metabolism and effects of selenium deficiency on thyroid hormone and iodine metabolism. *Biol. Trace Elem. Res.* **1992**, *34*, 321–325. [CrossRef] [PubMed]
72. Wesselink, E.; Koekkoek, W.A.C.; Grefte, S.; Witkamp, R.F.; van Zanten, A.R.H. Feeding mitochondria: Potential role of nutritional components to improve critical illness convalescence. *Clin. Nutr.* **2019**, *38*, 982–995. [CrossRef] [PubMed]

nutrients MDPI

Article

Erythrocyte Selenium as a Potential Key Indicator for Selenium Supplementation in Low-Selenium Populations: A Selenium Supplementation Study Based on Wistar Rats

Cunqi Lv [1,2,†], Ruixiang Wang [1,2,†], Qingyu Zeng [1,2], Chen Feng [1,2], Guijin Li [1,2], Shuxiu Hao [1,2], Jiacheng Li [1,2], Cheng Wang [1,2], Huixin Sun [1,2], Linlin Du [1,2], Yu Zhang [1,2], Xinshu Wang [3], Tong Wang [1,2,*] and Qi Li [4,*]

1 Institute of Keshan Disease, Chinese Center for Endemic Disease Control, Harbin Medical University, Harbin 150081, China; 2022020106@hrbmu.edu.cn (C.L.); 2020020149@hrbmu.edu.cn (R.W.)
2 Key Laboratory of Etiology and Epidemiology, Education Bureau of Heilongjiang Province (23618504) & Ministry of Health, Harbin Medical University, Harbin 150081, China
3 Department of Clinical Medicine, Queen Mary College, Nanchang University, Nanchang 330038, China
4 Department of Radiotherapy, Harbin Medical University Cancer Hospital, Harbin 150081, China
* Correspondence: wangtong@ems.hrbmu.edu.cn (T.W.); liqi@ems.hrbmu.edu.cn (Q.L.)
† These authors contributed equally to this work.

Abstract: Background: Selenium (Se) is an essential trace element for maintaining human health, with significant antioxidant and immunoregulatory functions. Inadequate Se intake may be associated with Keshan disease, Kashin–Beck disease, and hypothyroidism. However, effective indicators for scientifically guiding Se supplementation in Se-deficient populations are still lacking. Objectives: This study aims to explore the dynamic distribution of Se across various nutritional biomarkers and major organs in rats through a Se supplementation experiment, as well as the pairwise correlations between them, in order to identify reliable nutritional indicators for evaluating Se levels in the body. Methods: Se levels in hair, blood, and major tissues and organs were determined by atomic fluorescence spectrometry, and glutathione peroxidase (GSH-Px) levels were measured using an ELISA. Results: Se supplementation significantly increased Se levels in rat blood, hair, and major organs, as well as GSH-Px levels in blood. Se primarily accumulated in the liver and kidneys, followed by myocardium, spleen, and muscles. Serum and plasma Se were found to be the best indicators of short-term Se intake, while erythrocyte Se levels showed a stronger correlation with Se levels in tissues and organs, making it a better marker for assessing long-term Se nutritional status compared to hair Se. Conclusions: This study demonstrates the potential of erythrocyte Se levels as an indicator for evaluating long-term Se nutritional status, providing scientific evidence for Se nutritional assessments.

Keywords: nutritional status; erythrocyte selenium; serum selenium; hair selenium; glutathione peroxidase

1. Introduction

Selenium (Se) is an essential trace element for humans, playing a variety of critical physiological roles, including antioxidant, immunoregulatory, anti-inflammatory, anti-cancer, and anti-infection functions [1]. When Se concentrations are too low, its biological functions cannot be fully exerted [2], potentially increasing the risk of Keshan disease [3], Kashin–Beck disease, hypothyroidism, and miscarriage and other reproductive and obstetric complications [4,5]. Conversely, excessive Se intake may induce oxidative stress, leading to hair loss, nail deformities, neurological symptoms, and even life-threatening conditions [6–8].

Se nutritional status is commonly assessed by measuring Se levels in hair, plasma, and serum [9]. Hair Se levels are widely used to assess long-term Se intake due to the ease of sample collection, storage, transport, and high compliance [10]. Serum or plasma Se levels mainly reflect recent dietary Se intake [11]. Glutathione peroxidase (GSH-Px), known for its significant antioxidant properties, exhibits decreased activity during Se deficiency but recovers rapidly after Se supplementation. This makes it a common indicator of Se nutritional status and the body's antioxidant capacity [12].

Our previous study, which measured hair Se levels in 3026 residents across 28 provinces in China, found that 40.9% of the participants exhibited varying degrees of Se deficiency [10]. Dietary interventions and supplementation in Se-deficient areas have proven to be effective preventive measures [13]. However, given the narrow safety range of Se intake, uncontrolled long-term supplementation may lead to Se excess, posing potential health risks [14,15]. Due to economic constraints, sample preservation, transport, and technical limitations, it is challenging to comprehensively assess all Se nutritional indicators in practice. Therefore, identifying an efficient, stable, and representative biomarker to guide Se supplementation strategies is imperative.

Given this background, we conducted a Se supplementation experiment in Wistar rats to further explore the effects of Se supplementation on Se nutritional biomarkers (hair, whole blood, serum, plasma, erythrocyte, and GSH-Px), as well as Se levels in major tissues and organs (liver, kidneys, spleen, myocardium, and muscles). This study aims to explore the dynamic distribution of Se across various nutritional biomarkers and major organs in rats through a Se supplementation experiment, as well as the pairwise correlations between them, in order to identify reliable nutritional indicators for evaluating Se levels in the body.

2. Materials and Methods

2.1. Chemicals

Sodium selenite (SS) was purchased from Sigma-Aldrich (St. Louis, MO, USA).

2.2. Dosage Calculation

According to the guidelines for nutritional requirements, the recommended nutrient intake (RNI) for Se in humans is 55 μg/day, and the tolerable upper intake level (UL) is 400 μg/day [16]. To ensure the efficacy of the experiment without causing Se toxicity in rats, a human Se intake of 200 μg/day was used as the basis, assuming an average adult weight of 60 kg and applying a conversion factor (6.25) to account for animal tolerance [17]. The final dosage of SS for the rats was calculated to be 200 μg/L. Thus, a 200 μg/L SS solution was used for Se supplementation in the drinking water of the experimental group.

2.3. Selenium Supplementation Experiment in Rats

2.3.1. Animal Grouping and Sample Size

We strictly adhered to the 3R principles in determining the number of rats used in this study. The experiment is divided into five time phases, with sampling conducted once every seven days. For the control group, the minimum number of animals was maintained at five per stage, while in the selenium-supplemented (SS) group, the number was increased to 10 per stage to account for potential individual variability following supplementation. To prevent any impact from unforeseen losses, an additional 5 rats were included for the control group and 10 for the SS group. Additionally, to evaluate whether selenium levels in the control group changed significantly during the experiment compared to pre-experiment levels, a baseline group of 10 rats was established. Thus, the final composition included 10 rats in the baseline group, 30 in the control group, and 60 in the SS group, totaling 100 rats.

2.3.2. Animal Husbandry, Grouping, and Sampling Protocol for Selenium Supplementation Study in Wistar Rats

A total of 100 male Wistar rats, aged 6–8 weeks, were purchased from Beijing Vital River Laboratory Animal Technology Co., Ltd. (Beijing, China) and housed at the SPF-level Transgenic Animal Research Center of Harbin Medical University. The rats were kept in a

12 h light/dark cycle with free access to food and water. After a one-week acclimatization period, the rats were randomly divided into a baseline group (n = 10), an SS group (n = 60), and a control group (n = 30). The baseline group was sacrificed immediately, while the SS and control groups underwent a 5-week intervention. The SS group received drinking water supplemented with 200 μg/L SS (Se: 91.32 μg/L), while the control group received regular water (Se: 0 μg/L). There was no difference in the feed provided to the two groups of rats (Se: 0.15 mg/kg). Sampling points were taken every 7 days. In the first 4 weeks, 10 rats from the SS group and 5 from the control group were randomly selected and euthanized weekly. The remaining rats were sacrificed in the fifth week. Blood, hair, myocardium, liver, kidneys, spleen, and thigh muscles (the quadriceps muscles) were collected post-mortem. Hair samples (from the dorsum and ventral areas) were stored in polyethylene ziplock bags and kept in a dry, dark environment. Myocardium, liver, kidneys, spleen, and thigh muscles were weighed and stored along with whole blood, plasma, and serum samples in an ultra-low temperature freezer at −80 °C.

Blinding was applied throughout the processes of group assignment, housing, euthanasia, and relevant indicator assessments to ensure that the experimenters were unaware of the grouping conditions. The study strictly adhered to animal ethical standards and was approved by the Ethics Committee of the Center for Endemic Disease Control, Harbin Medical University (Approval No. hrbmuecdc20220402).

2.4. Organ Coefficient

The spleen, liver, kidney, and heart of the rats were excised and weighed. The relative weight of each organ was calculated based on the final body weight measured on the day of organ collection. The organ coefficients were calculated as follows:

$$\text{Organ coefficient (g/100 g)} = \text{organ weight/rat body weight} \times 100.$$

2.5. Measurement of Selenium Levels

Se levels were determined using an atomic fluorescence spectrometer (AFS 933, Beijing Titan Instrument Co., Beijing, China).

2.5.1. Sample Preparation

(1) Hair: 0.1 g of clean, dry hair samples were placed into 50 mL digestion vessels.

(2) Serum, plasma, and whole blood: 100 μL of each sample was placed into 50 mL conical flasks.

(3) Erythrocytes: Approximately 0.1 g of erythrocytes were weighed and placed into 50 mL conical flasks.

(4) Organs: Frozen myocardium, liver, kidneys, spleen, and thigh muscles were cut into small pieces, and approximately 0.1 g of each sample was placed into 50 mL conical flasks.

(5) Standard materials: Approximately 0.1 g of human hair reference material was weighed and placed into 50 mL conical flasks.

2.5.2. Determination of Selenium Levels in Samples

A mixture of 5 mL of acid (nitric acid and perchloric acid in a 4:1 ratio) was added to digest the samples or standard materials, which were left to stand overnight. The next day, thermal digestion was carried out at 180 °C using an electric sand bath. After cooling to room temperature, 5 mL of a hydrochloric acid solution (1:1 ratio of concentrated hydrochloric acid and deionized water) was added for reduction. Then, 1 mL of potassium ferricyanide solution was added, and the samples were diluted to 10 mL with 5% hydrochloric acid. Se levels were measured using the AFS-933 dual-channel atomic fluorescence spectrometer, and a standard curve was drawn based on Se content and fluorescence values. The blank samples, human hair reference material, and sample fluorescence values were measured sequentially. The Se content was determined using the standard curve. The recovery rate of Se was 88.8–117.1%.

2.6. Measurement of Glutathione Peroxidase (GSH-Px) Levels

GSH-Px levels in serum or plasma were measured using a GSH-Px assay kit (Jiancheng Biotech, Nanjing, China). Serum or plasma samples were diluted with physiological saline, and whole blood samples were prepared into hemolysates. Pre-experiments were conducted to determine the optimal dilution factor, ensuring an inhibition rate between 45% and 50%. Reagents were prepared according to the kit instructions, and GSH solutions and test samples were added to enzyme and non-enzyme tubes. The reaction was conducted in a 37 °C water bath. After the reaction, the supernatant was collected by centrifugation, and the samples were added to a microplate. Optical density (OD) values were measured at 405 nm using a microplate reader (BioTek Instruments, Winooski Charlotte, VT, USA).

2.7. Data Analysis

Data were analyzed using SPSS 17.0. The normality of the data was assessed using the Shapiro–Wilk test. For data that followed a normal or approximately normal distribution, the results were expressed as the mean ± standard deviation (SD), and group differences were analyzed using a *t*-test of independent samples. Spearman's rank correlation analysis was performed, with correlation coefficients represented by r_s. A *p*-value of <0.05 was considered statistically significant.

3. Results

3.1. Dietary Intake, Body Weight, and Organ Coefficients of Rats at Various Time Points

To identify the optimal indicator of Se nutritional status, we conducted a Se supplementation experiment in rats (Figure 1A). As shown in Figure 1B,C, the water intake and feed consumption levels of the rats were not significantly different between the control group and the SS group from the second to fifth week ($p > 0.05$), except in the first week, where the control group had a significantly higher intake than the SS group ($p < 0.01$). Further evaluation of the total Se intake from the diet (including feed and water), as shown in Figure 1D, revealed that the Se intake level in the SS group was significantly higher than that of the control group throughout the supplementation period ($p < 0.01$). The organ coefficients were assessed as shown in Figure 1E–I, and no significant differences in body weight or organ coefficients (liver, kidneys, spleen, heart) were observed between the SS rats and the control group at any time point during the supplementation period ($p > 0.05$). This suggests that Se supplementation had no significant impact on the body weight or the major organs of the rats.

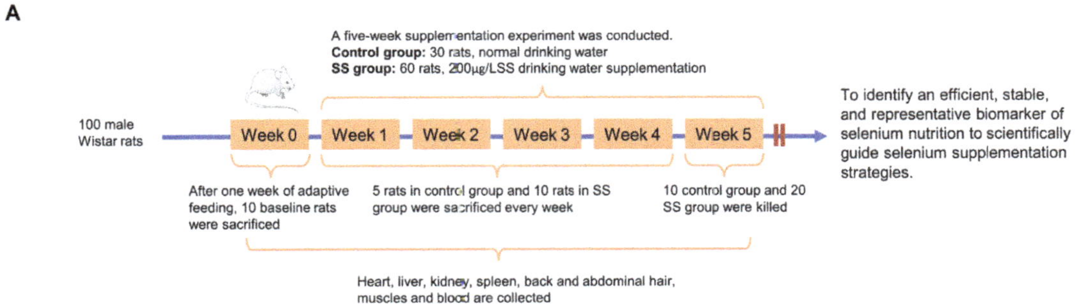

Figure 1. *Cont.*

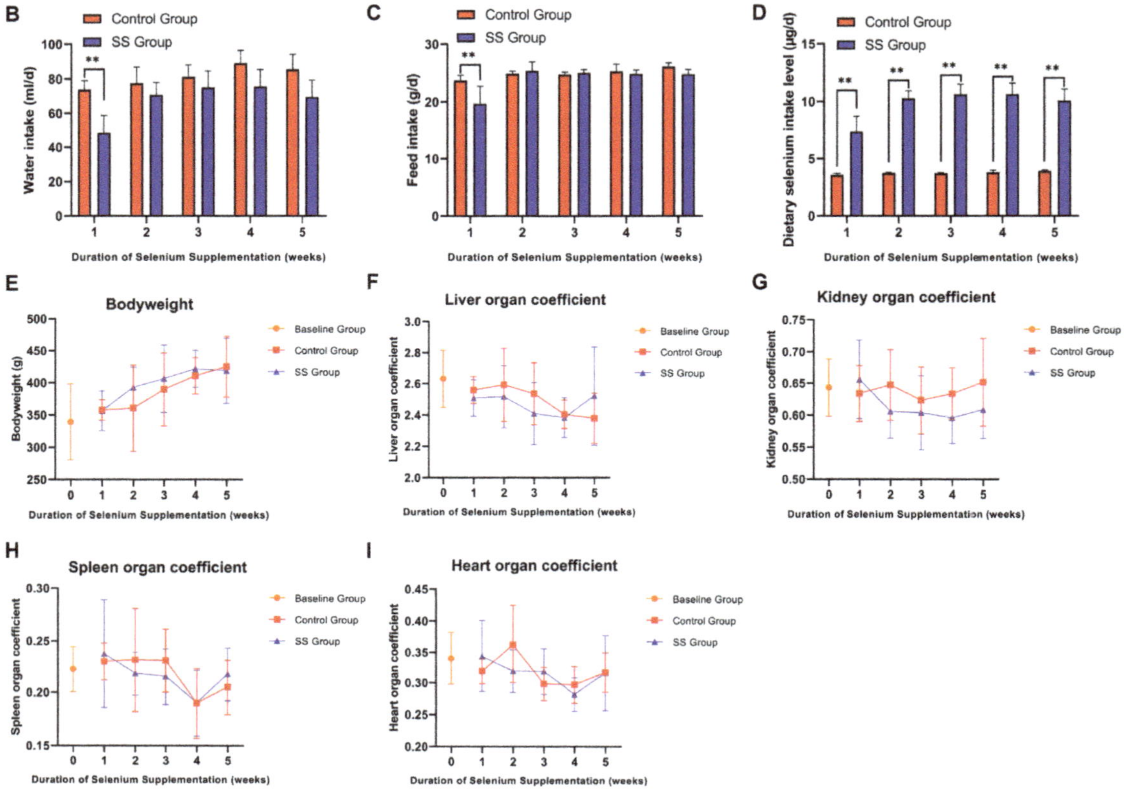

Figure 1. Dietary intake, body weight, and organ coefficients of rats in the control group and the Sodium selenite (SS) group at different time points. Flowchart of the selenium (Se) supplementation experiment in rats (**A**). Changes in water intake (**B**), feed intake (**C**), Se intake from diet (**D**), body weight (**E**), liver organ coefficient (**F**), kidney organ coefficient (**G**), spleen organ coefficient (**H**), and heart organ coefficient (**I**) at different time points. Asterisk indicates statistically significant differences between the SS group and the control group at corresponding time points, ** $p < 0.01$.

3.2. Selenium Nutritional Indicators in Rats at Various Time Points

To further explore the effect of Se supplementation on Se nutritional indicators in rats, we measured the Se levels in dorsal hair, ventral hair, whole blood, serum, plasma, and erythrocytes, along with GSH-Px levels in serum, plasma, and whole blood. As shown in Figure 2, the Se nutritional indicators in the control group rats did not exhibit significant fluctuations throughout the experimental period. In contrast, the Se nutritional indicators in the SS supplementation group showed varying degrees of increase compared to the control group ($p < 0.05$). Specifically, Se levels in dorsal hair, ventral hair, whole blood, and erythrocytes showed a continuous increase throughout the supplementation (Figure 2A–C,F). In contrast, serum and plasma Se levels increased sharply during the first week but plateaued over the subsequent weeks (Figure 2D,E). Additionally, GSH-Px levels in the serum, plasma, and whole blood samples showed a significant increase ($p < 0.05$). As the supplementation period progressed, GSH-Px levels continued rising; however, after the fourth week of supplementation, the increase was no longer statistically significant compared to the control group (Figure 2G–I).

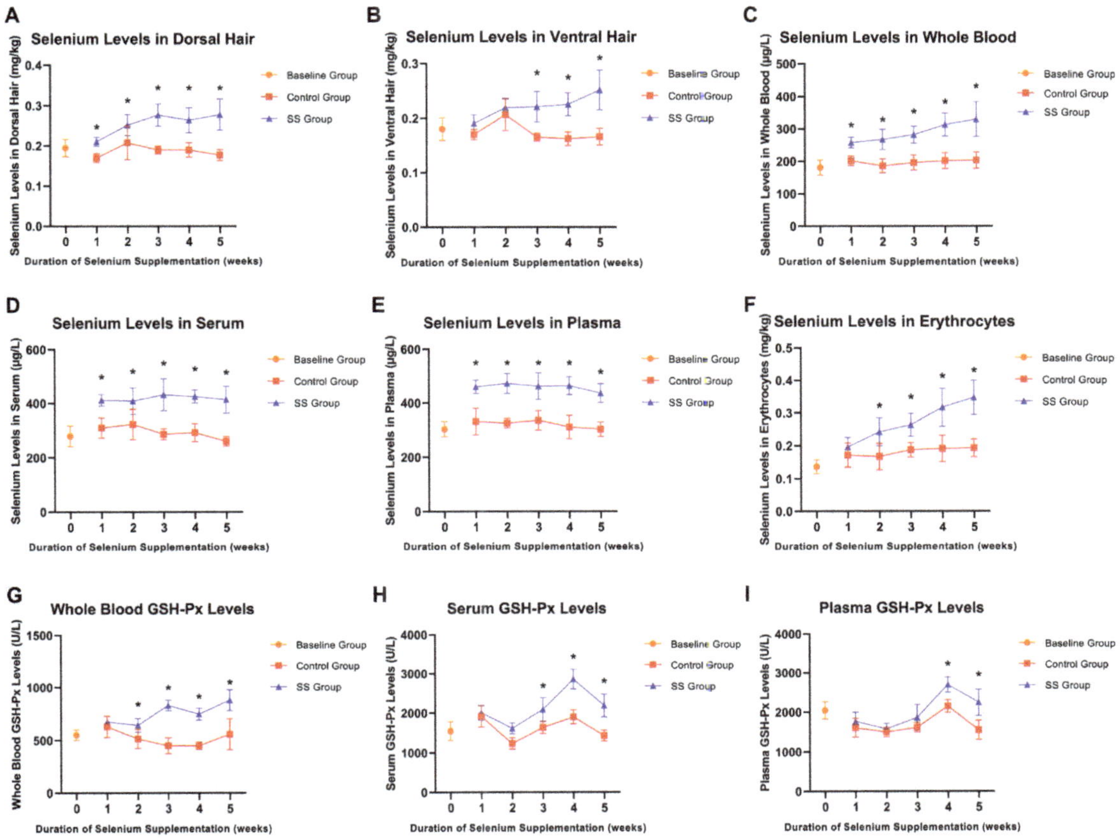

Figure 2. Changes in Se nutritional biomarkers in rats from the control group and SS group at different time points. Changes in dorsal hair Se (**A**), ventral hair Se (**B**), whole blood Se (**C**), serum Se (**D**), plasma Se (**E**), erythrocyte Se (**F**), whole blood GSH-Px (**G**), serum GSH-Px (**H**), and plasma GSH-Px (**I**) levels at different time points in rats. Asterisk indicates statistically significant differences in Se levels and GSH-Px activity between the SS group and the control group at corresponding time points, * $p < 0.05$.

3.3. Selenium Levels in Major Tissues and Organs of Rats at Various Time Points

To validate the impact of Se supplementation on the Se concentrations in major tissues and organs, we measured Se concentrations in the liver, kidneys, spleen, myocardium, and muscles. As shown in Figure 3, consistent with the Se nutritional indicators, the Se levels in the major tissues and organs of the control group did not exhibit significant changes. In contrast, the Se content in these organs significantly increased in the SS supplementation group, with a continuous upward trend as the supplementation period progressed.

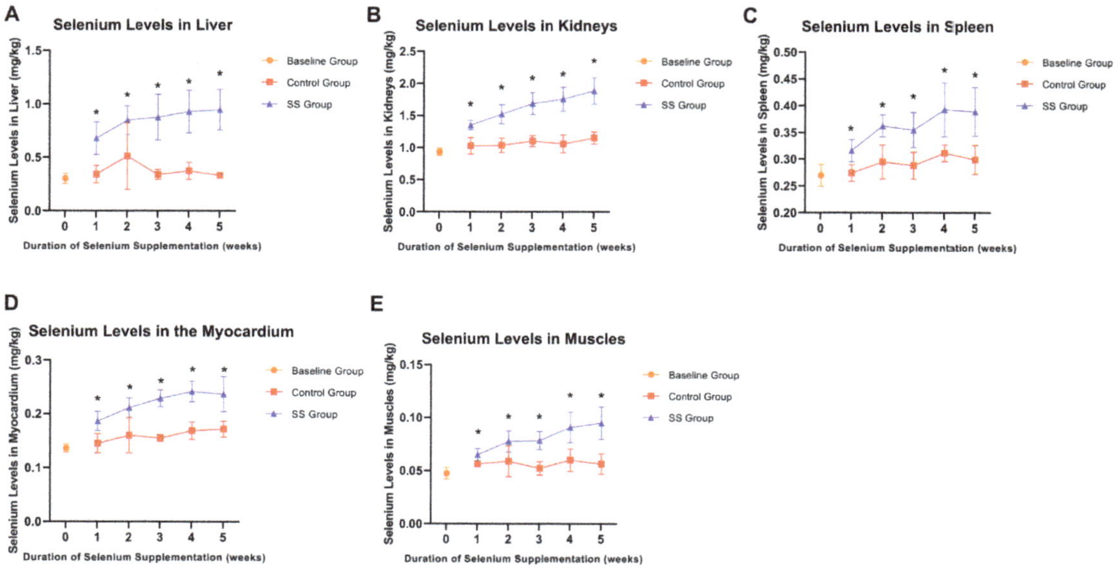

Figure 3. Changes in Se levels in various tissues and organs of rats from the control group and SS group at different time points. The Se level changes in liver (**A**), kidneys (**B**), spleen (**C**), myocardium (**D**), and muscles (**E**) at different time points in rats. Asterisk indicates statistically significant differences in Se levels between the SS group and the control group at the corresponding time points, * $p < 0.05$.

3.4. Selenium Enrichment in Nutritional Indicators and Major Organs

To assess Se accumulation in major organs, we evaluated the Se levels in the nutritional indicators and organs of rats after five weeks of supplementation, comparing them with the control group. As shown in Table 1, in the control group, Se was primarily concentrated in the kidneys, followed by the liver and spleen, with the lowest levels in the muscles. After five weeks of supplementation, while the kidneys remained the organ with the highest Se concentration, the liver showed the greatest fold change in Se accumulation (2.87), followed by the muscles (1.69) and the kidneys (1.63), with the smallest change observed in the spleen (1.30). Among the Se nutritional indicators, erythrocytes exhibited the highest fold change in Se accumulation (1.80), followed by whole blood Se (1.63) and serum Se (1.59).

Table 1. Se concentrations of biomarkers in rats from the control and SS groups.

Selenium Biomarkers	Control Group	SS Group	*t*-Value	*p*-Value	SS Group/ Control Group
Myocardial Selenium (mg/kg)	0.17	0.24	6.00	<0.0001	1.38
Muscle Selenium (mg/kg)	0.06	0.09	7.26	<0.0001	1.69
Spleen Selenium (mg/kg)	0.30	0.39	5.72	<0.0001	1.30
Liver Selenium (mg/kg)	0.33	0.95	10.16	<0.0001	2.87
Kidney Selenium (mg/kg)	1.16	1.89	10.75	<0.0001	1.63
Dorsal Hair Selenium (mg/kg)	0.18	0.28	7.92	<0.0001	1.57
Ventral Hair Selenium (mg/kg)	0.17	0.25	7.13	<0.0001	1.52
Whole Blood Selenium (μg/L)	203.08	330.41	6.74	<0.0001	1.63
Erythrocyte Selenium (mg/kg)	0.19	0.35	8.25	<0.0001	1.80
Plasma Selenium (μg/L)	302.48	436.65	10.63	<0.0001	1.44
Serum Selenium (μg/L)	259.85	413.92	8.89	<0.0001	1.59
Whole Blood GSH-Px (U/L)	556.34	877.06	6.97	<0.0001	1.58
Plasma GSH-Px (U/L)	1549.51	2243.05	5.83	<0.0001	1.45
Serum GSH-Px (U/L)	1427.55	2183.52	7.48	<0.0001	1.53

3.5. Correlation Analysis Between Selenium Nutritional Indicators and Major Organs

To explore the correlation between Se nutritional indicators and Se levels in major organs, we performed pairwise correlation analyses. As shown in Table 2, Se levels in the myocardium, liver, kidneys, spleen, and muscles exhibited strong intercorrelations with each other ($r_s > 0.8$). Further analysis revealed that whole blood and erythrocyte Se concentrations were highly correlated with Se levels in these organs ($r_s > 0.8$). In contrast, hair Se levels showed weaker correlations with organ Se levels, with correlation coefficients mostly ranging from 0.7 to 0.8. Additionally, GSH-Px levels in whole blood showed higher correlations with Se levels in the liver, kidneys, spleen, myocardium, and muscles ($0.6 < r_s < 0.8$) compared to serum and plasma Se levels ($0.3 < r_s < 0.7$).

Table 2. Correlation analysis of Se indicators in rats.

	Myocardial Se	Muscle Se	Spleen Se	Whole Blood Se	Liver Se	Kidney Se	Erythrocyte Se	Dorsal Hair Se	Ventral Hair Se	Plasma Se	Serum Se	Whole Blood GSH-Px	Plasma GSH-Px	Serum GSH-Px
Myocardial Se	1	0.877 **	0.834 **	0.843 **	0.868 **	0.890 **	0.838 **	0.816 **	0.721 **	0.706 **	0.726 **	0.741 **	0.415 **	0.602 **
Muscle Se		1	0.854 **	0.834 **	0.862 **	0.859 **	0.855 **	0.778 **	0.771 **	0.614 **	0.636 **	0.735 **	0.455 **	0.581 **
Spleen Se			1	0.779 **	0.835 **	0.810 **	0.830 **	0.732 **	0.718 **	0.613 **	0.606 **	0.688 **	0.436 **	0.536 **
Whole Blood Se				1	0.799 **	0.888 **	0.887 **	0.764 **	0.727 **	0.759 **	0.765 **	0.764 **	0.490 **	0.689 **
Liver Se					1	0.859 **	0.806 **	0.789 **	0.711 **	0.723 **	0.668 **	0.722 **	0.397 **	0.571 **
Kidney Se						1	0.897 **	0.803 **	0.716 **	0.696 **	0.706 **	0.788 **	0.405 **	0.623 **
Erythrocyte Se							1	0.738 **	0.708 **	0.612 **	0.634 **	0.736 **	0.486 **	0.614 **
Dorsal Hair Se								1	0.794 **	0.707 **	0.673 **	0.680 **	0.378 **	0.481 **
Ventral Hair Se									1	0.566 **	0.593 **	0.639 **	0.356 **	0.391 **
Plasma Se										1	0.820 **	0.593 **	0.263 **	0.535 **
Serum Se											1	0.651 **	0.374 **	0.626 **
Whole Blood GSH-Px												1	0.386 **	0.572 **
Plasma GSH-Px													1	0.763 **
Serum GSH-Px														1

Note: Asterisk indicates a statistically significant correlation coefficient, ** $p < 0.01$.

4. Discussion

In our previous cross-sectional study on Se nutritional levels in the Chinese population, we found that 40.9% of residents exhibited varying degrees of Se deficiency, with 5.3% experiencing severe deficiency [10]. Environmental factors and dietary habits are the primary determinants of human Se intake [18,19]. In China, insufficient dietary Se intake remains a significant challenge [8,20], particularly in low-Se regions, where Se deficiency disrupts the food chain and poses serious health risks to the population [21,22]. Research indicates that over 50% of Chinese children and 80% of elderly individuals consume dietary Se below the estimated average requirement level (EAR), highlighting the urgent need for Se supplementation in low-Se areas [23,24]. Therefore, a reliable Se nutritional indicator is needed to guide effective supplementation strategies.

As demonstrated in Figures 2 and 3, Se supplementation in rats significantly elevated Se levels in the liver, kidneys, spleen, myocardium, muscles, blood, and hair, while also enhancing GSH-Px activity. Serum and plasma Se levels reached saturation within the first week of supplementation, whereas Se levels in the hair, whole blood, erythrocytes, and major organs continued rising with extended supplementation. Serum and plasma Se levels remain important indicators for assessing short-term Se nutritional status, while erythrocyte and hair Se levels are more suitable for evaluating long-term Se nutritional status. Whole blood Se, which includes both plasma and erythrocyte Se, can comprehensively assess both long-term Se nutritional levels and short-term Se intake. These findings are consistent with the study by Solé-Navais et al. in Norway, which similarly concluded that whole blood Se concentration reflects both long-term status and short-term Se intake, while plasma/serum Se reflects only short-term status [25]. Moreover, studies by Costa and Stefanowicz confirmed that erythrocyte Se is less influenced by external factors, due to the longer lifespan of erythrocytes, making it a more accurate reflection of long-term Se nutritional status [26,27]. Although hair Se is often used to assess long-term nutritional status [3,28,29], its susceptibility to environmental factors and the potential reluctance of participants (e.g., women) to provide hair samples limit its utility as an indicator. GSH-Px, a Se-dependent antioxidant enzyme, plays a vital role in reducing oxidative stress and maintaining cellular redox balance, serving as a direct indicator of the body's antioxidant capacity [30,31]. In this study, Se supplementation significantly increased GSH-Px levels in rat blood, indicating an improvement in Se nutritional status. However, after four weeks of supplementation, GSH-Px levels plateaued, suggesting that the body had reached an optimal Se level, entering a state of Se nutritional balance. These results indicated that GSH-Px may serve as a useful biomarker for guiding Se supplementation strategies.

Our study also found that after five weeks of Se supplementation, Se levels in the liver and kidneys increased significantly, while the spleen and myocardium showed more moderate increases. The preferential accumulation of Se in the liver and kidneys is closely related to their roles in Se metabolism, storage, and excretion [32–34]. The liver is the primary site of selenoprotein synthesis, particularly for antioxidant enzymes like GSH-Px, which helps cells resist oxidative damage. The liver also distributes Se throughout the body in biologically active forms (e.g., SELENOP) [35]. Kidneys excrete excess Se, eliminating it in inorganic forms or Se metabolites via urine [36,37]. The relatively smaller changes in myocardial Se levels may be due to the myocardium's sensitivity to Se deficiency. Numerous studies have demonstrated a close association between selenium deficiency and cardiovascular diseases, with selenium deficiency increasing the risk of Keshan disease (endemic cardiomyopathy) [38], heart failure [39], and other cardiac disorders [40]. Liver and kidney function should be given close attention in future human Se supplementation studies to mitigate potential risks of damage.

Furthermore, Se levels show a high correlation among various organs and tissues. Among Se nutritional indicators, erythrocyte Se and whole blood Se had the highest correlation with Se levels in organs, followed by hair Se. Serum and plasma Se showed the weakest correlation, possibly because they reached saturation early in the supplementation process. In contrast, hair Se, due to its growth characteristics, may lag behind actual Se intake changes and be more influenced by environmental factors. Therefore, erythrocyte Se, compared to hair Se, is a more reliable indicator for evaluating long-term Se nutritional status. These findings provide scientific evidence for guiding future Se supplementation strategies in Se-deficient areas.

This study has several limitations. First, the exclusive use of male rats may introduce selection bias, as sex differences could influence the results. Additionally, we chose a 2:1 ratio of Se-supplemented rats to control rats to more comprehensively assess the effects of Se supplementation, rather than the traditional 1:1 ratio. Future research should validate the efficacy of erythrocyte Se as an indicator of long-term Se nutritional status using both male and female rats and more balanced group ratios to enhance the generalizability and applicability of the findings. Furthermore, this study only measured GSH-Px levels in whole blood, serum, and plasma, without evaluating GSH-Px levels in erythrocyte or other biomarkers reflecting the body's antioxidant capacity. In future studies, these additional parameters will be assessed to provide a more comprehensive evaluation of selenium's impact on the body's antioxidant function.

5. Conclusions

This study demonstrates that Se supplementation significantly increases Se levels in rat blood, hair, GSH-Px, liver, kidneys, spleen, myocardium, and muscles. Plasma and serum Se levels are important indicators for assessing short-term Se nutritional status, while erythrocyte Se is more effective for evaluating long-term Se nutritional status and proves to be more reliable than hair Se. The liver and kidneys are the primary sites of Se accumulation, both in the absence of and following supplementation. These findings provide critical scientific evidence to guide future Se supplementation strategies and optimize Se nutrition in deficient populations.

Author Contributions: Conceptualization, T.W. and Q.L.; methodology, C.L., R.W., T.W. and Q.L.; validation, C.L. and R.W.; formal analysis, C.F. and S.H.; investigation, C.L., R.W., Q.Z. and J.L.; data curation, G.L., C.W., Y.Z. and X.W.; writing—original draft preparation, C.L.; writing—review and editing, T.W. and C.L.; supervision, T.W.; supervision, L.D. and H.S.; project administration, T.W.; funding acquisition, T.W. All authors have read and agreed to the published version of the manuscript.

Funding: This study was supported by the National Natural Science Foundation of China (82073492).

Institutional Review Board Statement: The animal study protocol was approved by the Animal Ethics Committee of Harbin Medical University (hrbmuecdc20220402, 2 April 2024). Throughout the study, optimal husbandry conditions were maintained, and every effort was made to minimize the animals' suffering.

Informed Consent Statement: Not applicable.

Data Availability Statement: Data are contained within the article.

Acknowledgments: We acknowledge the financial support from the National Natural Science Foundation of China. This study used OpenAI's ChatGPT-4 v2 for partial grammar checking.

Conflicts of Interest: The authors declare that they have no known competing financial interests or personal relationships that could have appeared to influence the work reported in this paper.

References

1. Bjorklund, G.; Shanaida, M.; Lysiuk, R.; Antonyak, H.; Klishch, I.; Shanaida, V.; Peana, M. Selenium: An Antioxidant with a Critical Role in Anti-Aging. *Molecules* **2022**, *27*, 6613. [CrossRef] [PubMed]
2. Chen, N.; Yao, P.; Zhang, W.; Zhang, Y.; Xin, N.; Wei, H.; Zhang, T.; Zhao, C. Selenium nanoparticles: Enhanced nutrition and beyond. *Crit. Rev. Food Sci. Nutr.* **2023**, *63*, 12360–12371. [CrossRef] [PubMed]
3. Liu, H.; Yu, F.; Shao, W.; Ding, D.; Yu, Z.; Chen, F.; Geng, D.; Tan, X.; Lammi, M.J.; Guo, X. Associations Between Selenium Content in Hair and Kashin-Beck Disease/Keshan Disease in Children in Northwestern China: A Prospective Cohort Study. *Biol. Trace Elem. Res.* **2018**, *184*, 16–23. [CrossRef] [PubMed]
4. Mistry, H.D.; Broughton Pipkin, F.; Redman, C.W.; Poston, L. Selenium in reproductive health. *Am. J. Obstet. Gynecol.* **2012**, *206*, 21–30. [CrossRef] [PubMed]
5. Rayman, M.P.; Wijnen, H.; Vader, H.; Kooistra, L.; Pop, V. Maternal selenium status during early gestation and risk for preterm birth. *CMAJ* **2011**, *183*, 549–555. [CrossRef]
6. Naderi, M.; Puar, P.; Zonouzi-Marand, M.; Chivers, D.P.; Niyogi, S.; Kwong, R.W.M. A comprehensive review on the neuropathophysiology of selenium. *Sci. Total Environ.* **2021**, *767*, 144329. [CrossRef]
7. Zhang, F.; Li, X.; Wei, Y. Selenium and Selenoproteins in Health. *Biomolecules* **2023**, *13*, 799. [CrossRef]
8. Gorini, F.; Sabatino, L.; Pingitore, A.; Vassalle, C. Selenium: An Element of Life Essential for Thyroid Function. *Molecules* **2021**, *26*, 7084. [CrossRef]
9. Müller, S.M.; Dawczynski, C.; Wiest, J.; Lorkowski, S.; Kipp, A.P.; Schwerdtle, T. Functional Biomarkers for the Selenium Status in a Human Nutritional Intervention Study. *Nutrients* **2020**, *12*, 676. [CrossRef]
10. Jia, Y.; Wang, R.; Li, G.; Feng, C.; Qi, L.; Wang, Y.; Su, S.; Zou, Y.; Liu, X.; Wang, Y.; et al. Hair Selenium of Residents in Keshan Disease Endemic and Non-endemic Regions in China. *Biol. Trace Elem. Res.* **2023**, *201*, 3256–3267. [CrossRef]
11. Urbano, T.; Filippini, T.; Wise, L.A.; Sucato, S.; Polledri, E.; Malavolti, M.; Fustinoni, S.; Michalke, B.; Vinceti, M. Selenium exposure and urinary 8-oxo-7,8-dihydro-2′-deoxyguanosine: Major effects of chemical species and sex. *Sci. Total Environ.* **2023**, *870*, 161584. [CrossRef] [PubMed]
12. Rogulska, J.; Osowska, S.; Kunecki, M.; Sobocki, J.; Ładyżyński, P.; Giebułtowicz, J. Antioxidant balance in plasma of patients on home parenteral nutrition: A pilot study comparing three different lipid emulsions. *Clin. Nutr.* **2021**, *40*, 3950–3958. [CrossRef] [PubMed]
13. Rayman, M.P. Selenium and human health. *Lancet* **2012**, *379*, 1256–1268. [CrossRef]
14. Ferro, C.; Florindo, H.F.; Santos, H.A. Selenium Nanoparticles for Biomedical Applications: From Development and Characterization to Therapeutics. *Adv. Healthc. Mater.* **2021**, *10*, e2100598. [CrossRef]
15. Little, M.; Achouba, A.; Ayotte, P.; Lemire, M. Emerging evidence on selenoneine and its public health relevance in coastal populations: A review and case study of dietary Se among Inuit populations in the Canadian Arctic. *Nutr. Res. Rev.* 2024, 1–10, *Online ahead of print*. [CrossRef]
16. Peng, S.; Zhang, G.; Wang, D. Association of selenium intake with bone mineral density and osteoporosis: The national health and nutrition examination survey. *Front. Endocrinol.* **2023**, *14*, 1251838. [CrossRef]
17. Li, Q.; Li, T.; Cao, X.C.; Luo, D.Q.; Lian, K.J. Methylprednisolone microsphere sustained-release membrane inhibits scar formation at the site of peripheral nerve lesion. *Neural Regen. Res.* **2016**, *11*, 835–841.
18. Zhang, Y.; Meng, S.; Yu, Y.; Bi, L.; Tian, J.; Zhang, L. Associations of dietary selenium intake with the risk of chronic diseases and mortality in US adults. *Front. Nutr.* **2024**, *11*, 1363299. [CrossRef]
19. Navarro-Alarcon, M.; Cabrera-Vique, C. Selenium in food and the human body: A review. *Sci. Total Environ.* **2008**, *400*, 115–141. [CrossRef]

20. Liu, T.; Liu, X.; Zhou, R.; Chen, H.; Zhang, H.; Zhang, B. De novo Transcriptome Assembly and Comparative Analysis Highlight the Primary Mechanism Regulating the Response to Selenium Stimuli in Oats (*Avena sativa* L.). *Front. Plant Sci.* **2021**, *12*, 625520. [CrossRef]
21. Zhao, X.; Lu, Y.; Dai, L.; Wang, L.; Zhou, G.; Liang, T. Selenium spatial distribution and bioavailability of soil-plant systems in China: A comprehensive review. *Environ. Geochem. Health* **2024**, *46*, 341. [CrossRef] [PubMed]
22. Wang, X.; Li, H.; Yang, L.; Kong, C.; Wang, J.; Li, Y. Selenium Nutritional Status of Rural Residents and Its Correlation with Dietary Intake Patterns in a Typical Low-Selenium Area in China. *Nutrients* **2020**, *12*, 3816. [CrossRef] [PubMed]
23. Liu, Z.; Zhao, L.; Man, Q.; Wang, J.; Zhao, W.; Zhang, J. Dietary Micronutrients Intake Status among Chinese Elderly People Living at Home: Data from CNNHS 2010–2012. *Nutrients* **2019**, *11*, 1787. [CrossRef]
24. Wang, H.; Wang, D.; Ouyang, Y.; Huang, F.; Ding, G.; Zhang, B. Do Chinese Children Get Enough Micronutrients? *Nutrients* **2017**, *9*, 397. [CrossRef]
25. Solé-Navais, P.; Brantsæter, A.L.; Caspersen, I.H.; Lundh, T.; Muglia, L.J.; Meltzer, H.M.; Zhang, G.; Jacobsson, B.; Sengpiel, V.; Barman, M. Maternal Dietary Selenium Intake during Pregnancy Is Associated with Higher Birth Weight and Lower Risk of Small for Gestational Age Births in the Norwegian Mother, Father and Child Cohort Study. *Nutrients* **2020**, *13*, 23. [CrossRef]
26. Costa, N.A.; Gut, A.L.; Pimentel, J.A.; Cozzolino, S.M.; Azevedo, P.S.; Fernandes, A.A.; Polegato, B.F.; Tanni, S.E.; Gaiolla, R.D.; Zornoff, L.A.; et al. Erythrocyte selenium concentration predicts intensive care unit and hospital mortality in patients with septic shock: A prospective observational study. *Crit. Care* **2014**, *18*, R92. [CrossRef]
27. Stefanowicz, F.A.; Talwar, D.; O'Reilly, D.S.; Dickinson, N.; Atkinson, J.; Hursthouse, A.S.; Rankin, J.; Duncan, A. Erythrocyte selenium concentration as a marker of selenium status. *Clin. Nutr.* **2013**, *32*, 837–842. [CrossRef]
28. Lemire, M.; Mergler, D.; Huel, G.; Passos, C.J.; Fillion, M.; Philibert, A.; Guimarães, J.R.; Rheault, I.; Borduas, J.; Normand, G. Biomarkers of selenium status in the Amazonian context: Blood, urine and sequential hair segments. *J. Expo. Sci. Environ. Epidemiol.* **2009**, *19*, 213–222. [CrossRef]
29. Thomson, C.D. Assessment of requirements for selenium and adequacy of selenium status: A review. *Eur. J. Clin. Nutr.* **2004**, *58*, 391–402. [CrossRef]
30. Lai, C.Y.; Cheng, S.B.; Lee, T.Y.; Hsiao, Y.F.; Liu, H.T.; Huang, Y.C. Impact of Glutathione and Vitamin B-6 in Cirrhosis Patients: A Randomized Controlled Trial and Follow-Up Study. *Nutrients* **2020**, *12*, 1978. [CrossRef]
31. Sun, L.; Wang, F.; Wu, Z.; Ma, L.; Baumrucker, C.; Bu, D. Comparison of Selenium Source in Preventing Oxidative Stress in Bovine Mammary Epithelial Cells. *Animals* **2020**, *10*, 842. [CrossRef] [PubMed]
32. Erkekoglu, P.; Arnaud, J.; Rachidi, W.; Kocer-Gumusel, B.; Favier, A.; Hincal, F. The effects of di(2-ethylhexyl) phthalate and/or selenium on trace element levels in different organs of rats. *J. Trace Elem. Med. Biol.* **2015**, *29*, 296–302. [CrossRef] [PubMed]
33. Zhu, M.L.; Gao, Z.T.; Lu, J.X.; Wang, Y.; Wang, G.; Zhu, T.T.; Li, P.; Liu, C.; Wang, S.X.; Yang, L. Amorphous nano-selenium quantum dots prevent pulmonary arterial hypertension through recoupling endothelial nitric oxide synthase. *Aging* **2020**, *13*, 3368–3385. [CrossRef] [PubMed]
34. Mehdi, Y.; Dufrasne, I. Selenium in Cattle: A Review. *Molecules* **2016**, *21*, 545. [CrossRef]
35. Schwarz, M.; Meyer, C.E.; Löser, A.; Lossow, K.; Hackler, J.; Ott, C.; Jäger, S.; Mohr, I.; Eklund, E.A.; Patel, A.A.H.; et al. Excessive copper impairs intrahepatocyte trafficking and secretion of selenoprotein P. *Nat. Commun.* **2023**, *14*, 3479. [CrossRef]
36. Yanjun, Y.; Jing, Z.; Yifei, S.; Gangzhao, G.; Chenxin, Y.; Qiang, W.; Qiang, Y.; Shuwen, H. Trace elements in pancreatic cancer. *Cancer Med.* **2024**, *13*, e7454. [CrossRef]
37. Khatiwada, S.; Subedi, A. A Mechanistic Link Between Selenium and Coronavirus Disease 2019 (COVID-19). *Curr. Nutr. Rep.* **2021**, *10*, 125–136. [CrossRef]
38. Li, C. Selenium deficiency and endemic heart failure in China: A case study of biogeochemistry for human health. *Ambio* **2007**, *36*, 90–93. [CrossRef]
39. Metes-Kosik, N.; Luptak, I.; Dibello, P.M.; Handy, D.E.; Tang, S.S.; Zhi, H.; Qin, F.; Jacobsen, D.W.; Loscalzo, J.; Joseph, J. Both selenium deficiency and modest selenium supplementation lead to myocardial fibrosis in mice via effects on redox-methylation balance. *Mol. Nutr. Food Res.* **2012**, *56*, 1812–1824. [CrossRef]
40. Weening, E.H.; Al-Mubarak, A.A.; Dokter, M.M.; Dickstein, K.; Lang, C.C.; Ng, L.L.; Metra, M.; van Veldhuisen, D.J.; Touw, D.J.; de Boer, R.A.; et al. Sexual dimorphism in selenium deficiency is associated with metabolic syndrome and prevalence of heart disease. *Cardiovasc. Diabetol.* **2023**, *22*, 8. [CrossRef]

nutrients

MDPI

Article

Alleviation of Lipid Disorder and Liver Damage in High-Fat Diet-Induced Obese Mice by Selenium-Enriched *Cardamine violifolia* with Cadmium Accumulation

Junying Zhu [1,†], Qingqing Lv [1,†], Fengna Li [1,†], Ping Xu [1], Ziyu Han [1], Aolin Yang [1], Zhan Shi [1], Chao Wang [2], Jie Jiang [2], Yunfen Zhu [3], Xiaofei Chen [3], Lvhui Sun [4], Xin Gen Lei [5,*] and Ji-Chang Zhou [1,6,7,*]

1 School of Public Health (Shenzhen), Shenzhen Campus of Sun Yat-sen University, Shenzhen 518107, China; zhujy85@mail2.sysu.edu.cn (J.Z.); lvqq6@mail2.sysu.edu.cn (Q.L.); lifengn@mail2.sysu.edu.cn (F.L.); xuping8@mail2.sysu.edu.cn (P.X.); hanzy8@mail2.sysu.edu.cn (Z.H.); yangaolin@mail2.sysu.edu.cn (A.Y.); shizh28@mail2.sysu.edu.cn (Z.S.)

2 Shenzhen Center for Disease Control and Prevention, Shenzhen 518055, China; raulw2003@163.com (C.W.); szjiangjie@139.com (J.J.)

3 Enshi Autonomous Prefecture Academy of Agricultural Sciences, Enshi 445000, China; azhu19@163.com (Y.Z.); chenxiaofei_05@163.com (X.C.)

4 Hubei Hongshan Laboratory, College of Animal Science and Technology, Huazhong Agricultural University, Wuhan 430070, China; lvhuisun@mail.hzau.edu.cn

5 Department of Animal Science, Cornell University, Ithaca, NY 14853, USA

6 Guangdong Province Engineering Laboratory for Nutrition Translation, Shenzhen 518107, China

7 Guangdong Provincial Key Laboratory of Food, Nutrition and Health, Guangzhou 510080, China

* Correspondence: xl20@cornell.edu (X.G.L.); zhoujch8@mail.sysu.edu.cn (J.-C.Z.)

† These authors contributed equally to this work.

Abstract: Background/Objectives: As a hyperaccumulator of selenium (Se), *Cardamine violifolia* (*Cv*) and its peptide extract could ameliorate the negative effects of a high-fat diet (HFD). However, the effects of the coaccumulation of cadmium (Cd) in Se-enriched *Cv* (*Cv2*) and the potential confounding effect on the roles of enriched Se remain unknown. We aimed to investigate whether *Cv2* could alleviate HFD-induced lipid disorder and liver damage. Methods: Three groups of 31-week-old female mice were fed for 41 weeks (n = 10–12) with a control *Cv*-supplemented diet (*Cv1*D, 0.15 mg Se/kg, 30 μg Cd/kg, and 10% fat calories), a control *Cv*-supplemented HFD (*Cv1*HFD, 45% fat calories), and a *Cv2*-supplemented HFD (*Cv2*HFD, 1.5 mg Se/kg, 0.29 mg Cd/kg, and 45% fat calories). Liver and serum were collected to determine the element concentrations, markers of liver injury and lipid disorder, and mRNA and/or protein expression of lipid metabolism factors, heavy metal detoxification factors, and selenoproteins. Results: Both *Cv1*HFD and *Cv2*HFD induced obesity, and *Cv2*HFD downregulated Selenoi and upregulated Dio3 compared with *Cv1*D. When comparing *Cv2*HFD against *Cv1*HFD, *Cv2* increased the liver Se and Cd, the protein abundance of Selenoh, and the mRNA abundance of 10 selenoproteins; reduced the serum TG, TC, and AST; reduced the liver TG, lipid droplets, malondialdehyde, and mRNA abundance of *Mtf1* and *Mt2*; and differentially regulated the mRNA levels of lipid metabolism factors. Conclusions: *Cv2* alleviated HFD-induced lipid dysregulation and liver damage, which was probably associated with its unique Se speciation. However, further research is needed to explore the interaction of plant-coenriched Se and Cd and its effects on health.

Keywords: obesity; metabolic disorder; selenoprotein; heavy metal

1. Introduction

As one of the trace essential elements for both humans and animals, selenium (Se) serves as a critical and unique constitutive part of selenocysteine (Sec) in 25 human and 24 rodent selenoproteins [1]. Both organic and inorganic forms of Se from external sources can be efficiently absorbed via the gastrointestinal tract. Organic forms of Se generally exhibit lower toxicity, higher bioavailability, and better antioxidant properties than inorganic forms [2]. Plants can serve as carriers of beneficial elements for the maintenance of body health and are major sources of Se supplementation, as they are capable of biotransforming selenate and selenite into organic Se forms [3].

Cardamine violifolia (*Cv*) is a medicinal and edible plant, characterized by being a hyper-accumulator of Se [4]. Moreover, by enriching Se in the major forms of selenocystine and methylselenocystine [5], Se-enriched *Cv* is being developed as a promising Se-rich source. Concerningly, soils in Se-rich areas in the Enshi region of China often contain high levels of cadmium (Cd) [6,7]. In addition to Se, *Cv* could also accumulate the harmful heavy metal Cd [8], and the accumulation of Cd by *Cv* increases with the level of Se fertilization [8,9], thus yielding Se-enriched *Cv* (*Cv2*). The most common type of Cd exposure in non-smoking populations occurs through food and water contaminated with Cd [10], and Cd continuously accumulates in tissue due to the absence of effective excretory mechanisms. As exemplified by the severe Cd poisoning-induced itai-itai disease [11], the long-term accumulation of Cd can eventually cause damage to the functions of various organs in the body, including the liver, kidneys, bones, testes, and others [12]. Interestingly, recent studies have shown that *Cv2*-derived endogenous Se has the potential to antagonize Cd-induced renal damage, skeletal metabolism disorders, and hepatotoxicity [8,9]. Furthermore, reports of Cd-related toxicity are uncommon in areas with high geologic backgrounds of Se and Cd, which may be attributed to the interaction between Se and Cd in plants, leading to alterations in the forms of Cd present in plants that enter the human body, thereby reducing the toxicity of Cd [13,14]. On the other hand, Se can partially alleviate the body health damage caused by Cd exposure [14,15].

It is important to note that obesity has also progressively become one of the most important public health problems in the world [16] and is a significant risk factor for the development and progression of multiple diseases, such as type 2 diabetes, hypertension, hyperlipidemia, non-alcoholic fatty liver disease, and immune disorders [17–19]. Many animal studies have found that Se plays a beneficial role in improving lipid metabolic disorder and liver damage [20–22], and *Cv*-derived Se-enriched peptides (CSP) could alleviate those phenotypes induced by a high-fat diet (HFD) [23]. However, combined exposure to a HFD and Cd often results in stronger toxic effects on the body [24–26], while the effect of Se in the presence of plant-derived Cd accumulation on the adverse health consequences induced by a HFD in Se–Cd-rich areas remains unknown.

Thus, by applying *Cv2* to feed adult female mice with varied dietary fat for more than 40 weeks, our study was to investigate the effect of *Cv2*-derived endogenous Se, in the presence of Cd accumulation, on the lipid metabolic disorders and liver injuries caused by the long-term exposure to HFD. Additionally, we hope to provide some new insights into the effects of Se on ameliorating adverse effects of HFD and Cd caused by consuming foods in naturally Se–Cd-rich areas.

2. Materials and Methods

2.1. Diets and Animals

The control *Cv* (*Cv1*) and *Cv2* powders used in this study were provided by the Enshi Academy of Agricultural Sciences. Regarding the cultivation methods and conditions of *Cv*, briefly, *Cv1* was cultivated in soil with Se and Cd concentrations of 1.22 mg/kg and 0.61 mg/kg, respectively. On a field adjacent to that for *Cv1* planting, during the same season, *Cv2* was obtained by cultivating the same strain of *Cv1* with Se fertilizer-treated soil (Enshi Zhonghui Selenium Enriched Agricultural Technology Development Co., Ltd., Enshi, China) at a concentration of $\geq$200 mg Se/kg and with sodium selenite (purity of 97%) applied through foliar spraying. After the two types of whole plants were harvested, they were rinsed, dried, ground, and sieved to obtain a *Cv1* powder (total Se: 7.24 mg/kg; total Cd: 1.4 mg/kg) and a *Cv2* powder (total Se: 76.95 mg/kg; total Cd: 14.5 mg/kg). Over 80% of the Se in these powders existed in the forms of selenocystine and methylselenocystine [5].

The three types of feed used during the experiment were prepared by the Trophic Animal Feed High-Tech Co., Ltd., Nantong, China. For the Se-deficient diet used in all three types of feed, except for Se, all components of this diet met the standards of AIN93.

The *Cv1* powder was supplemented into the Se-deficient diet to contain 0.15 mg Se/kg and 0.03 mg Cd/kg, with fat providing 10% or 45% of the energy, to obtain the *Cv1*-supplemented control diet (*Cv1*D) or the *Cv1*-supplemented HFD (*Cv1*HFD), respectively. The *Cv2* powder was used to replace the same amount of *Cv1* powder in *Cv1*HFD to obtain the *Cv2*-supplemented HFD (*Cv2*HFD), containing 1.5 mg Se/kg and 0.29 mg Cd/kg.

All animal experiments reported in this manuscript were approved by the Animal Care and Use Committee of the Institute of Sun Yat-sen University and adhered to the criteria outlined in the 'Guide of the Care and Use of Laboratory Animals'. Thirty-four female C57BL/6J mice aged 31 weeks, purchased from the Guangdong Medical Laboratory Animal Center, were randomly divided into three groups and fed *Cv1*D (n = 12), *Cv1*HFD (n = 12), and *Cv2*HFD (n = 10) based on the baseline body weight (BW). The animals were maintained under standard conditions, including 4–5 mice per cage, a temperature of 25 ± 2 °C, 70–75% humidity, and a light/dark cycle of 12 h, with free access to food and water during the experimentation. The experimental period was 41 weeks, and the BW was monitored every four weeks for each mouse. At the end of the experiment, all mice were fasted overnight and anesthetized with sodium pentobarbital to minimize pain before being euthanized by heart bleeding.

2.2. Oral Glucose Tolerance Test (OGTT) and Insulin Tolerance Test (ITT)

At the 40th week of the animal experiment, all mice were fasted for 6 h. Tail vein blood glucose was measured with a glucometer (ACCU-CHEK Performa, Roche Diagnostics GmbH, Mannheim, Germany). The OGTT was performed using an oral gavage of 2 g/kg BW of glucose, and blood glucose was measured at 0, 15, 30, 60, and 120 min after glucose loading. In the middle of the 41st week of the experiment, all mice were fasted for 4 h. Then, the ITT was performed using an intraperitoneal injection of 1 U/kg BW of insulin, and blood glucose was measured at 0, 15, 30, 60, 90, and 120 min after insulin loading with a glucometer. Prior to measuring the tail vein blood glucose and administering insulin via intraperitoneal injection, mild and non-irritating disinfection with an iodine tincture was performed on the local area to minimize animals' pain and stress and to reduce the risk of infection.

2.3. Sample Preparation and Biochemical Analysis

Blood and tissue samples were collected promptly for analysis or cryopreservation. The serum samples were isolated by centrifugation at 12,000× g for 10 min at 4 °C. Approximately 50 mg liver samples were homogenized and centrifugated at 2500× g for 10 min at 4 °C to collect the supernatant. For the prepared serum and liver homogenate samples, commercial kits were used to measure the concentrations of TG (Fujifilm Wako Pure Chemical Co., Osaka, Japan), total cholesterol (TC), and low-density lipoprotein cholesterol (LDL-C) (Nanjing Jiancheng Bioengineering Institute, Nanjing, China). The serum activity of alanine aminotransferase (ALT) and aspartate transaminase (AST) was measured by a HITACHI Automatic Analyzer 3100 at the Laboratory Animal Center of Sun Yat-sen University.

2.4. Elemental Analysis

Element quantification in the *Cv1*, *Cv2*, *Cv1*D, *Cv1*HFD, *Cv2*HFD, and liver tissue was performed using an Agilent 7850 Inductively Coupled Plasma Mass Spectrometer (Agilent Technologies, Santa Clara, CA, USA). Briefly, for sample digestion using an oven, 5 mL of nitric acid was added to a fluoroplastic liner containing an individual sample, and the samples in the insert were pre-incubated for 30 min at 80 °C. Subsequently, they were incubated for 2 h at 110 °C, followed by an additional incubation step for 4 h at 160 °C. Then, the dissolved samples were allowed to cool down to room temperature and quantitatively transferred to test tubes. Finally, a specific volume of deionized water was added to the test tubes, which were then vortexed and further assayed.

2.5. Malondialdehyde (MDA) Levels and Total Antioxidant Capacity (T-AOC)

To analyze the MDA levels, 20 mg liver samples were homogenized with phosphate-buffered saline using a tissue grinder. The homogenate was centrifuged at 3000× g for

10 min at 4 °C, and the supernatant was collected for analysis using an MDA assay kit (Nanjing Jiancheng Bioengineering Institute, Nanjing, China). For T-AOC measurement, the liver homogenate was centrifuged at 12,000× *g* for 5 min at 4 °C. Then, the supernatant was collected for analysis using a T-AOC assay kit (Nanjing Jiancheng Bioengineering Institute, Nanjing, China).

2.6. Histological Analysis

Six mice were randomly selected from each group and the histopathology of hepatic steatosis was evaluated by determining the average number, size, and area of hepatic lipid droplets. The freshly isolated livers of the mice were fixed in 10% neutral buffered formalin and then embedded in paraffin and sliced at 5 µm. After this, sections of the liver were stained with hematoxylin and eosin (H&E). The quantitative analysis of the number and size of the lipid droplets was performed using the ImageJ software 1.52v with three fields per slide, and the mean values were calculated.

2.7. RNA Extraction and Quantitative Real-Time PCR (qPCR)

Total RNA was extracted from the liver tissue using a total RNA extraction reagent (Yeasen Biotech (Shanghai) Co., Ltd., Shanghai, China), according to the manufacturer's instructions. The concentration and purity of the RNA were determined by measuring the absorbance at 260/280 nm using a spectrophotometer (NanoDrop, Thermo Fisher Scientific, Waltham, MA, USA). The RNA integrity was checked by agarose gel electrophoresis. cDNA was synthesized using a reverse transcription kit (Takara Biomedical Technology (Beijing) Co., Ltd., Beijing, China), and then qPCR was performed. All primers for the selenoprotein genes and lipid metabolism-related genes used in the qPCR are listed in Table S1. Relative quantification was performed using the $2^{-\Delta\Delta CT}$ method normalized to the control *Actb*.

2.8. Western Blot Assay

The Western blotting experiment was performed according to a protocol previously described [27]. Briefly, 20 mg liver samples were homogenized in ice-cold RIPA lysis buffer (Beyotime Biotechnology, Shanghai, China) containing complete protease inhibitor using a tissue grinder. The homogenate was centrifuged at 12,000× *g* for 15 min at 4 °C, and the supernatant was collected. The protein concentration was determined using the BCA Protein Assay Kit (Thermo Fisher Scientific). After this, equal amounts of protein (usually 20 µg) from each sample were separated by SDS-PAGE and transferred onto a PVDF membrane (0.22 or 0.45 µm, Millipore, Burlington, MA, USA). Then, the membrane was blocked with 5% non-fat milk in a Tris–Tween-buffered saline buffer (TBST) for 2 h and was incubated with primary antibodies (Table S2) overnight at 4 °C. After washing with TBST, the membrane was incubated with horseradish peroxidase-conjugated secondary antibodies (dilution: 1:5000) for 1 h at room temperature. Finally, blots were developed on the membrane using Mini-ChemiTM910 reagents (Beijing SinSage Technology Co., Ltd., Beijing, China). We digitally quantified the resultant signals and normalized the data to the Actb abundance.

2.9. Statistical Analysis

All data were presented as the mean ± SEM. Statistical analysis was performed using GraphPad Prism 9.51 (GraphPad Software Inc., San Diego, CA, USA) and SPSS 26.0 (SPSS Inc., Chicago, IL, USA). The differences between the groups were determined using one-way or two-way ANOVA with Tukey's multiple comparison test. The results were considered statistically significant at $p < 0.05$.

3. Results

3.1. Growth Performance

Over the 41 weeks of HFD administration, we found that *Cv2* did not significantly alleviate HFD-induced weight gain in female mice. As shown in Figure 1, there was no significant difference in BW between the *Cv1*HFD and *Cv2*HFD groups ($p \geq 0.05$).

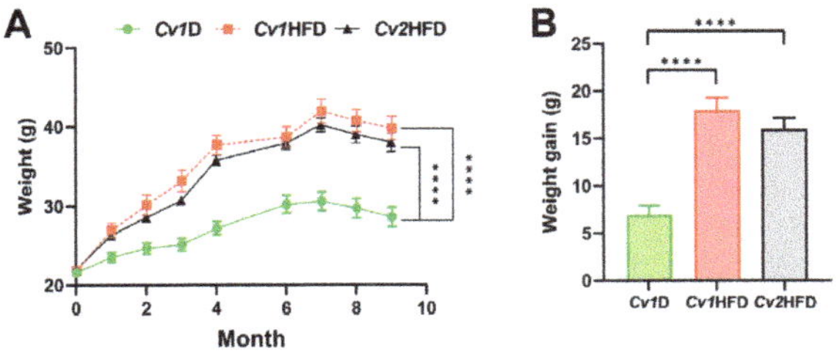

Figure 1. Growth performance in adult female mice during the 41-week experiment. (**A**) Body weight. (**B**) Total weight gain. Data are means ± SEM (n = 10–12) and differ with ****, $p < 0.0001$. *Cv1*D, control diet with 0.15 mg Se and 0.03 mg Cd (in the form of control *Cv*)/kg; *Cv*, *Cardamine violifolia*; *Cv1*HFD, high-fat diet with 0.15 mg Se and 0.03 mg Cd (in the form of control *Cv*)/kg; *Cv2*HFD, high-fat diet with 1.5 mg Se and 0.29 mg Cd (in the form of Se-enriched *Cv*)/kg.

3.2. Concentrations of Trace Elements in the Liver

Compared with those of the *Cv1*D or *Cv1*HFD group, the accumulation of Se significantly increased by ~22% in the livers of the *Cv2*HFD group ($p < 0.0001$; Figure 2A), while the accumulation of Cd significantly increased by 360% or 500%, respectively ($p < 0.0001$; Figure 2B). However, there was no difference in either Se or Cd between the *Cv1*D and *Cv1*HFD groups ($p \geq 0.05$). We also observed a significant association between the Se and Cd levels in the *Cv1*D group ($R^2 = 0.4822$, $p = 0.0379$) and all mice ($R^2 = 0.5612$, $p < 0.0001$; Figure 2C). Furthermore, no differences were observed in the concentrations of copper, iron, and zinc among the *Cv1*D, *Cv1*HFD, and *Cv2*HFD groups ($p \geq 0.05$; Figure S1A–C).

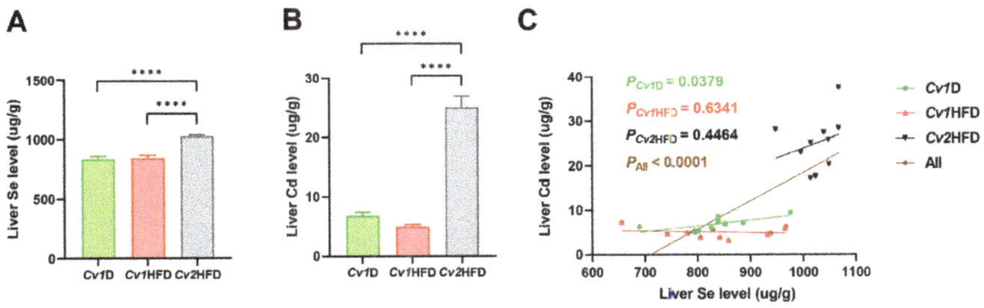

Figure 2. Accumulation of selenium (Se) (**A**) and cadmium (Cd) (**B**) and their correlation (**C**) in the livers of adult female mice. Data are means ± SEM (n = 9–12) and differ with ****, $p < 0.0001$. *Cv1*D, control diet with 0.15 mg Se and 0.03 mg Cd (in the form of control *Cv*)/kg; *Cv*, *Cardamine violifolia*; *Cv1*HFD, high-fat diet with 0.15 mg Se and 0.03 mg Cd (in the form of control *Cv*)/kg; *Cv2*HFD, high-fat diet with 1.5 mg Se and 0.29 mg Cd (in the form of Se-enriched *Cv*)/kg.

3.3. Glucose Metabolism

After the mice were fasted for 12 h before the OGTT test, the blood glucose levels in the *Cv1*HFD group and *Cv2*HFD group were both significantly higher than those in the *Cv1*D group at 60 min ($p < 0.05$; Figure S2A). Interestingly, although differences were not observed at other time points or in the glucose area under the curve (AUC) of OGTT among the three groups, there was a trend toward lower blood glucose levels in the *Cv2*HFD group compared with the *Cv1*HFD group (Figure S2B). For the ITT assessment, the fast plasma glucose level and the blood glucose level at 30 min after the injection of insulin in the mice in the *Cv1*HFD and *Cv2*HFD groups were significantly higher than those in the *Cv1*D group ($p < 0.05$; Figure S2C). However, no difference in the glucose AUC was observed among the three groups ($p \geq 0.05$; Figure S2D).

3.4. Lipid Disorder and Liver Injury

Compared with the *Cv1*HFD group, *Cv2* significantly decreased the serum levels of TG (20%, $p < 0.05$; Figure 3A) and TC (210%, $p < 0.05$; Figure 3B), as well as liver TG (59%, $p < 0.05$; Figure 3D), in the *Cv2*HFD group, without a significant effect on the serum LDL-C ($p \geq 0.05$; Figure 3C) and liver TC and LDL-C ($p \geq 0.05$; Figure 3E,F). Furthermore, although no difference was observed in the serum ALT activity ($p \geq 0.05$; Figure 3G), *Cv2* alleviated HFD-induced liver injuries, characterized by a ~33% decrease in serum AST activity in the *Cv2*HFD group compared with the *Cv1*HFD group ($p < 0.05$; Figure 3H).

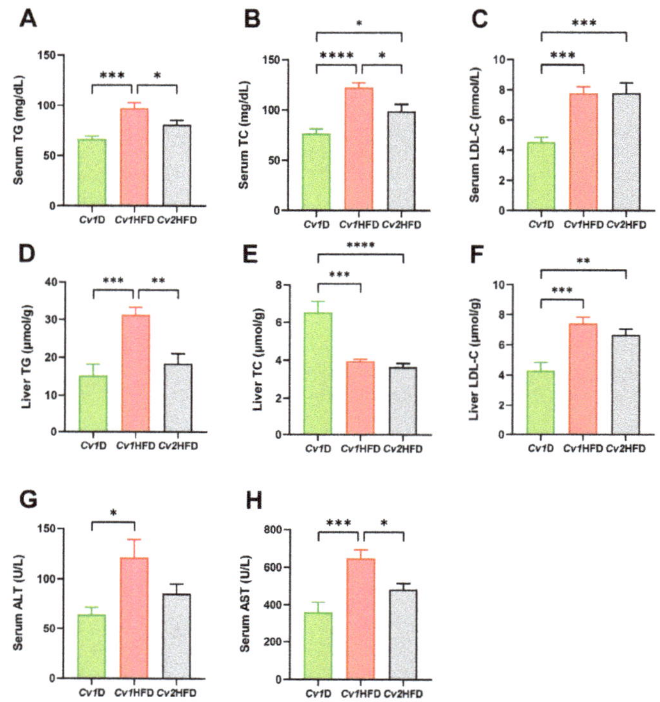

Figure 3. Lipid levels in the serum and liver and hepatic injury in adult female mice. (**A–C**) Serum concentrations of TG, TC, and LDL-C. (**D–F**) Liver concentrations of TG, TC, and LDL-C. (**G**,**H**) Serum ALT and AST activity. Data are means ± SEM (n = 8–10) and differ with *, $p < 0.05$; **, $p < 0.01$; ***, $p < 0.001$; and ****, $p < 0.0001$. ALT, alanine aminotransferase; AST, aspartate transaminase; *Cv1*D, control diet with 0.15 mg Se and 0.03 mg Cd (in the form of control *Cv*)/kg; *Cv*, *Cardamine violifolia*; *Cv1*HFD, high-fat diet with 0.15 mg Se and 0.03 mg Cd (in the form of control *Cv*)/kg; *Cv2*HFD, high-fat diet with 1.5 mg Se and 0.29 mg Cd (in the form of Se-enriched *Cv*)/kg; LDL-C, low-density lipoprotein cholesterol; Se, selenium; TC, total cholesterol; TG, triglyceride.

3.5. Regulating Gene and Protein Expression in Lipid Metabolism

In the *Cv1*HFD group, unclear intercellular boundaries, shrinking nuclei squeezed to the edges of the cell, and the disordered arrangement of hepatic cords were observed (Figure 4A). In the *Cv2*HFD group, hepatic lipid droplets were significantly fewer and smaller, with clearer boundaries of liver cells than those in the *Cv1*HFD group ($p < 0.05$). However, there was no significant difference in the liver weight among the *Cv1*D, *Cv1*HFD, and *Cv2*HFD groups ($p \geq 0.05$; Figure 4B).

The mRNA levels of key genes (*Gpat1*, *Gpat2*, *Dgat1*, and *Dgat2*) involved in TG synthesis showed no significant differences in the livers of *Cv1*HFD-fed female mice compared with *Cv1*D-fed female mice ($p \geq 0.05$), but a gene involved in TG hydrolysis

(*Lipc*) was significantly downregulated ($p < 0.05$; Figure 4C). In contrast, in the livers of *Cv*2HFD-fed mice, genes involved in TG synthesis (*Gpat1* and *Dgat2*) and genes involved in TG hydrolysis (*Atgl* and *Hsl*) were significantly downregulated compared to the *Cv*1HFD group, while the mRNA levels of *Lipc* and *Lpl* were significantly upregulated ($p < 0.05$).

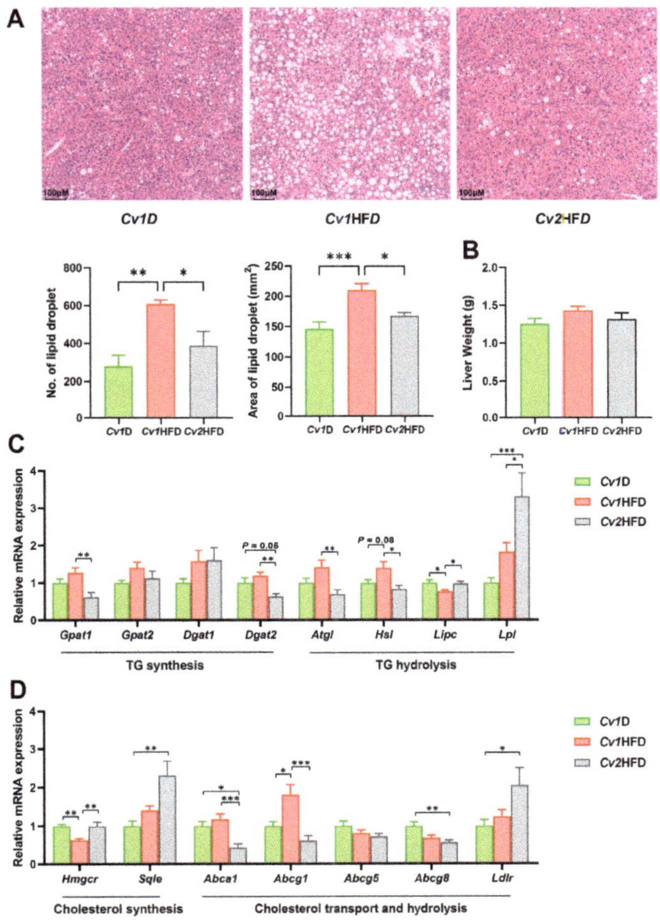

Figure 4. Improvement due to selenium (Se)-enriched *Cardamine violifolia* (*Cv*) in hepatic lipid accumulation and related molecular mechanisms. (**A**) H&E staining of the liver tissue with scale bar = 100 μM; the average number and area of hepatic lipid droplets were quantified with three fields per slide by using the "Analyze particles" function of ImageJ, and the mean values were calculated. (**B**) Total liver weight. (**C**) Expression of metabolic genes of triglycerides. (**D**) Expression of metabolic genes of cholesterol. Data are means ± SEM (n = 6–12) and differ with *, $p < 0.05$; **, $p < 0.01$; and ***, $p < 0.001$. *Abca1*, ATP-binding cassette subfamily A member 1; *Abcg1/5/8*, ATP-binding cassette subfamily G member 1/5/8; *Atgl*, adipose triglyceride lipase; ATP, adenosine triphosphate; *Cv*1D, control diet with 0.15 mg Se and 0.03 mg Cd (in the form of control *Cv*)/kg; *Dgat1/2*, diacylglycerol O-acyltransferase 1/2; *Gpat1/2*, glycerol-3-phosphate acyltransferase 1/2; *Cv*1HFD, high-fat diet with 0.15 mg Se and 0.03 mg Cd (in the form of control *Cv*)/kg; *Cv*2HFD, high-fat diet with 1.5 mg Se and 0.29 mg Cd (in the form of Se-enriched *Cv*)/kg; *Hmgcr*, 3-hydroxy-3-methylglutaryl coenzyme A reductase; *Hsl*, hormone-sensitive lipase; *Ldlr*, low-density lipoprotein receptor; *Lipc*, lipase C hepatic type; *Lpl*, lipoprotein lipase; No., number; *Sqle*, squalene epoxidase.

Regarding cholesterol homeostasis in the livers of *Cv1*HFD-fed mice, a key gene involved in cholesterol synthesis, *Hmgcr*, was significantly downregulated compared to *Cv1*D-fed mice, and a gene involved in cholesterol transport, *Abcg1*, was upregulated ($p < 0.05$; Figure 4D). In the livers of *Cv2*HFD-fed mice, the mRNA levels of *Hmgcr*, *Sqle*, and *Ldlr* were significantly upregulated compared to the *Cv1*HFD and/or *Cv1*D group(s), while the mRNA levels of *Abca1*, *Abcg1*, and *Abcg8* were significantly downregulated ($p < 0.05$).

3.6. Hepatic Oxidative Stress and Antioxidant Defense Capacity

Compared with those of the *Cv1*HFD group, *Cv2* significantly downregulated the elevated mRNA expression levels of metal regulatory transcription factor 1 (*Mtf1*) and metallothionein 2 (*Mt2*) caused by the HFD in the livers of the *Cv2*HFD group ($p < 0.05$; Figure 5A,C). Furthermore, no differences in the relative protein levels of Mtf1, Mt, and Sod1, as well as the T-AOC level, were observed among the *Cv1*D, *Cv1*HFD, and *Cv2*HFD groups ($p \geq 0.05$; Figure 5E–H). However, we found that, compared with the *Cv1*HFD group, *Cv2* significantly decreased the liver MDA level in the *Cv2*HFD group by ~75% ($p < 0.05$; Figure 5I).

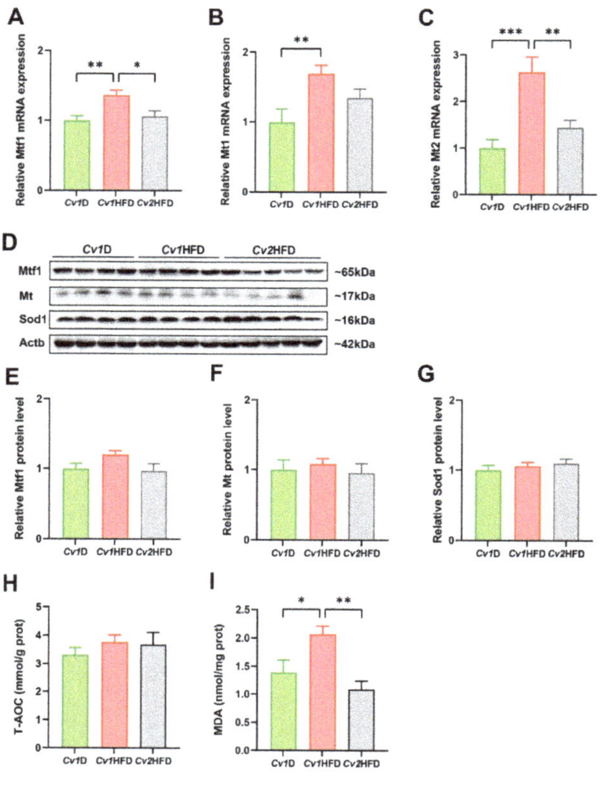

Figure 5. Oxidative stress and antioxidant levels in the livers of adult female mice. (**A–C**) The relative mRNA expression of *Mtf1*, *Mt1*, and *Mt2*. (**D**) A representative immunoblot image for Mtf1, Mt, and Sod1. (**E–G**) The relative protein levels of Mtf1, Mt, and Sod1. (**H**) The T-AOC level. (**I**) The level of MDA in the liver. Data are means ± SEM (n = 8–12) and differ with *, $p < 0.05$; **, $p < 0.01$; and ***, $p < 0.001$. *Cv1*D, control diet with 0.15 mg Se and 0.03 mg Cd (in the form of control *Cv*)/kg; *Cv*, *Cardamine violifolia*; *Cv1*HFD, high-fat diet with 0.15 mg Se and 0.03 mg Cd (in the form of control *Cv*)/kg; *Cv2*HFD, high-fat diet with 1.5 mg Se and 0.29 mg Cd (in the form of Se-enriched *Cv*)/kg; MDA, malondialdehyde; *Mt1/2*, metallothionein 1/2; *Mtf1*, metal regulatory transcription factor 1; Se, selenium; Sod1, superoxide dismutase 1; T-AOC, total antioxidant capacity.

3.7. Relative mRNA and Protein Expression of Selenoproteins

The mRNA abundance of all selected selenoprotein genes showed no differences ($p \geq 0.05$) between the *Cv1*D and *Cv1*HFD groups (Figure 6A,B; Figure S3). However, compared with those in the *Cv1*D and/or *Cv1*HFD group(s), the expression of 12 selenoprotein genes (*Dio1*, *Dio3*, *Gpx4*, *Msrb1*, *Selenof*, *Selenoo*, *Selenos*, *Selenow*, *Sephs2*, *Txnrd1*, *Txnrd2*, and *Txnrd3*) was significantly upregulated, while *Selenoi* was significantly downregulated in the livers of the *Cv2*HFD group ($p < 0.05$; Figure 6A,B).

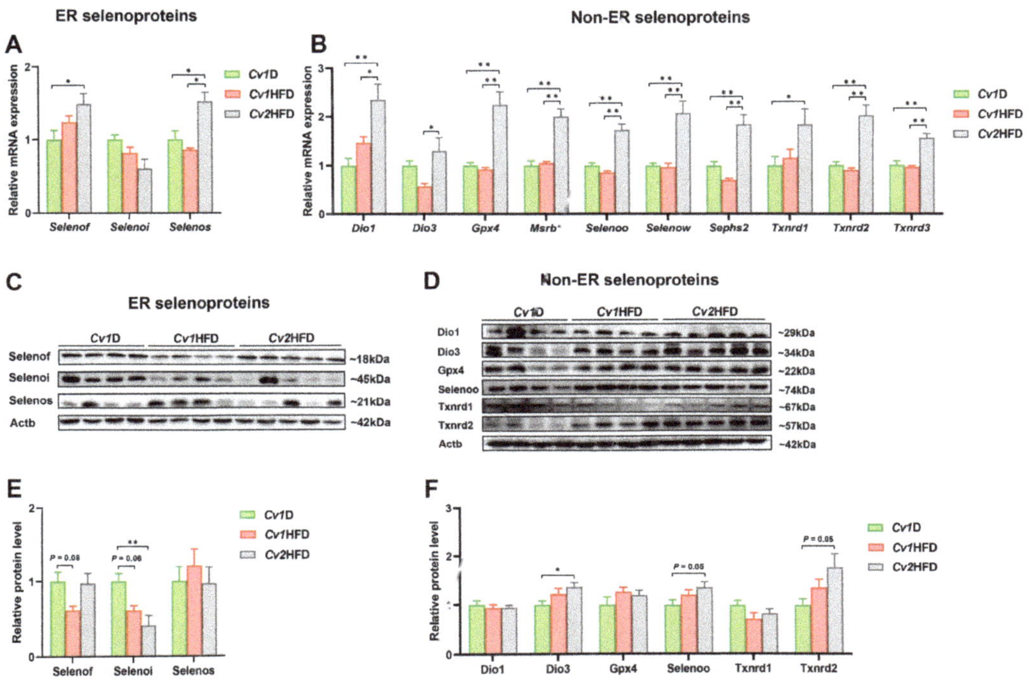

Figure 6. Expression of selenoproteins in the livers of adult female mice. (**A**) The relative mRNA expression levels of *Selenof*, *Selenoi*, and *Selenos*. (**B**) The relative mRNA expression levels of *Dio1*, *Dio3*, *Gpx4*, *Msrb1*, *Selenoo*, *Selenow*, *Sephs2*, *Txnrd1*, *Txnrd2*, and *Txnrd3*. (**C**) A representative immunoblot image for Selenof, Selenoi, and Selenos. (**D**) A representative immunoblot image for Dio1, Dio3, Gpx4, Selenoo, Txnrd1, and Txnrd2. (**E**) The relative protein levels of Selenof, Selenoi, and Selenos. (**F**) The relative protein levels of Dio1, Dio3, Gpx4, Selenoo, Txnrd1, and Txnrd2. Data are means ± SEM (n = 8–12) and differ with *, $p < 0.05$ and **, $p < 0.01$. *Cv1*D, control diet with 0.15 mg Se and 0.03 mg Cd (in the form of control *Cv*)/kg; *Cv*, *Cardamine violifolia*; *Dio1/3*, iodothyronine deiodinase 1/3; ER, endoplasmic reticulum; *Gpx4*, glutathione peroxidase 4; *Cv1*HFD, high-fat diet with 0.15 mg Se and 0.03 mg Cd (in the form of control *Cv*)/kg; *Cv2*HFD, high-fat diet with 1.5 mg Se and 0.29 mg Cd (in the form of Se-enriched *Cv*)/kg; *MsrB1*, methionine sulfoxide reductase B1; Se, selenium; *Selenof/i/o/s/w*, selenoprotein F/I/O/S/W; *Sephs2*, selenophosphate synthetase 2; *Txnrd1/2/3*, thioredoxin reductase 1/2/3.

Compared with those of the *Cv1*D group, the relative protein levels of the ER-resident Selenoi and the non-ER-resident Dio3 were, respectively, downregulated and upregulated in the livers of the *Cv2*HFD group ($p < 0.05$; Figure 6C–F). Furthermore, compared with those of the *Cv1*HFD group, the relative protein level of Selenoh was upregulated in the livers of the *Cv2*HFD group ($p < 0.05$; Figure S3C,D). Although there were no differences in the relative protein levels of Selenoo and Txnrd2 among the *Cv1*D, *Cv1*HFD, and *Cv2*HFD groups, there was an upregulatory trend in the *Cv2*HFD group ($p = 0.05$).

4. Discussion

The potential of Se-rich plants as a source for the development of novel Se supplements has drawn attention from many researchers due to their ability to improve health [23,28,29]. *Cv*, as a hyperaccumulator of Se, serves as an ideal plant-derived Se source. Previous studies have found that CSP from *Cv* may alleviate HFD-induced disorder of lipid metabolism through potential mechanisms such as increased thermogenesis and reduced oxidative stress and inflammation, as well as the regulation of gene expression in lipid and cholesterol metabolism [23]. However, *Cv* is also able to hyperaccumulate Cd, which hinders its promotion as an ideal Se supplement and calls for further investigations of the health effects of Se–Cd coenrichment in this species, as well as other plants [14,15]. Zhang et al. [8,9] aquacultured three types of Se–Cd-coenriched *Cvs* by supplementing 0, 1, or 2 mg/L of sodium selenate and 35 mg/L of cadmium chloride ($CdCl_2$) in the culturing solution and found that both Se (0.2–0.86 g/kg) and Cd (4.2–5.4 g/kg) in *Cv* positively increased with the Se supplementation. By gavage in mice with a purified water control or the same dosage of Cd (3.2 mg/kg BW) in the form of $CdCl_2$ or any of the three Se–Cd-coenriched *Cvs*, the Cd-induced renal damage, skeletal metabolism disorder [9], and hepatotoxicity [8] were improved with the increased Se levels across the three Se–Cd-coenriched *Cvs*, in which selenocystine probably played a critical role.

Given the characteristic of *Cv* being able to accumulate Se and Cd, we observed the naturally increased enrichment of Cd from the soil with Se supplementation in our study, which was consistent with the findings from other studies [7,8]. In our studied animals, the Cd exposure levels were much lower than those reported to cause significant liver damage [8,9,24,30–33]. Additionally, in the intervention model, the Se/Cd ratio (1.5 mg/kg Se vs. 0.29 mg/kg Cd) in our study was 5.17, while, in other studies showing the protective effect of Se against Cd exposure, the ratios were 0.16 (0.5 mg/kg Se vs. 3.2 mg/kg Cd) [8,9] and 0.8 (1.6 mg/kg Se vs. 2 mg/kg Cd) [34], much lower than ours. Se supplementation has been shown to improve the adverse health effects induced by HFD or Cd exposure; however, combined exposure to Cd and HFD often exhibits a synergistic effect in terms of damage to the health of the body [24,33,35]. Meanwhile, the role of Se in the presence of Cd accumulation on long-term HFD-induced health outcomes remains unknown. Thus, we conducted this study to investigate the effects of *Cv2* on metabolic disorder and liver damage induced by the long-term consumption of a HFD and to explore the role of Se in the plant-derived high background of Cd.

We found that, despite the tenfold increase in both the Se and Cd levels in *Cv2*HFD compared to *Cv1*D and *Cv1*HFD, there was a significant difference in the accumulation levels of Se and Cd in the livers. Indeed, under physiological conditions, there is a mechanism in the body to maintain Se homeostasis, primarily regulated through urinary excretion rather than absorption [36]. However, mammals lack effective regulatory mechanisms to control the balance of Cd levels in the body. Thus, the small amount of Cd entering the body through food or other pathways could be excreted in minute quantities through the urine, with the majority continuously accumulating in organs like the liver and eventually causing harm to the body [37]. Previous studies have revealed that combined exposure to a HFD and Cd could significantly disrupt the essential metal homeostasis in female mice, which could be associated with influencing the expression of metal transporters [24]. However, this phenomenon was not observed in our study. This could be explained by Se being capable of alleviating the effect of the HFD and Cd in terms of disrupting essential metal homeostasis by regulating metal transporters to some extent [24,38]. It is well known that a long-term HFD can disrupt lipid metabolism, leading to obesity, lipid metabolic disorder, and liver damage [39,40]. Furthermore, chronic low Cd exposure (150 μg/L $CdCl_2$ or 92 μg/L Cd spiked in pure water) at food limitation-relevant levels is sufficient to cause significantly disrupted hepatic energy metabolism homeostasis [41]. Therefore, the presence of Cd in *Cv2* may influence the protective effect of Se against the metabolic disorder induced by a long-term HFD, potentially exacerbating the health damage in synergy with the HFD. Although we found that *Cv2* did not significantly influence glucose tolerance or insulin sensitivity in HFD-induced female obese mice, we observed that the supplementation of *Cv2* could alleviate the increase in serum and hepatic lipid levels, as well as liver injury marker levels, induced by the HFD in mice, which may be attributed to the protective effects of *Cv*-derived endogenous Se on lipid metabolic disorder and liver injury induced by a HFD and Cd [23,29,42].

Lipid disorder is closely associated with abnormalities in lipid (including TG and TC) synthesis, transport, and metabolism. Previous studies have found that Cd can downregulate the expression of Atgl and Lpl [43], while, in HFD-fed mice, CSP increased the expression of Lpl and reduced the expression of Hmgcr [23]. Similarly, another study also demonstrated that, in normal diet-fed broilers, Se-enriched *Cv* could upregulate the expression of LPL and reduce the expression of HMGCR in the liver, without an effect on DGAT2. Obviously, Se, Cd, and HFD could affect lipid homeostasis by influencing the expression of lipid metabolism-related factors. In our study, *Cv2* downregulated the gene expression of TG synthesis enzymes (*Gpat1* and *Dgat2*) and upregulated TG hydrolytic enzymes (*Lipc* and *Lpl*), which are helpful in alleviating the HFD-induced elevation of TG levels [44]. Interestingly, some results in our study differed from previous research. We observed that the expression of the other two TG hydrolytic enzyme genes (*Atgl* and *Hsl*) was downregulated by *Cv2* supplementation in HFD-fed mice. Furthermore, we observed that *Cv2* upregulated *Hmgcr* in the *Cv2*HFD group compared with the *Cv1*HFD group. These findings, differing from previous research, suggest that the plant-derived Cd accumulation in the mouse liver affected Se's antagonistic effect on the HFD. We also observed that *Cv2* reduced the expression of cholesterol transport-related genes (*Abca1*, *Abcg1*) while increasing the expression levels of *ldlr* involved in cholesterol clearance in the *Cv2*HFD group, which are helpful in reducing cholesterol efflux and promoting its clearance [45]. This might have contributed to the lower serum TC level in the *Cv2*HFD group than in the *Cv1*HFD group [45–47]. Therefore, although its effectiveness was attenuated by the presence of plant-derived Cd, the endogenous Se in *Cv2* still demonstrated beneficial improvements in lipid metabolic disorder in HFD-induced obese mice.

Mts, particularly Mt1 and Mt2, are widely present in the parenchymal organs, such as the liver and kidneys, of mice, while Mtf1 serves as a positive regulatory factor for the expression of *Mts* [48,49]. They mainly participate in the detoxification of heavy metals, free radical scavenging, and protection against oxidative damage and are capable of inhibiting the toxicity of Cd [49]. Consistent with previous studies, we observed the upregulation of the gene expression levels of *Mtf1*, *Mt1*, and *Mt2* in the mouse liver induced by *Cv1*HFD; this may be a response of the body to HFD-induced oxidative stress [50,51]. Furthermore, we found that *Cv2* supplementation reduced the expression of these genes. Previous studies have found that exposure to Cd could upregulate the expression of *Mtf1*, *Mt1*, and *Mt2*, while Se reversed this effect [52], and the observed phenomenon between the *Cv1*HFD and *Cv2*HFD groups in our study may be attributed to the antagonistic effects of Se against Cd and the HFD. However, we observed no difference in the relative protein levels of Mt and Mtf1 among the three groups. In fact, a study also found that a HFD significantly increased the mRNA expression of *Mt2*, and the protein expression levels of Mts showed no significant difference compared to the control group [24], while another study reported the opposite results [33]. In fact, Mts primarily participate in maintaining the homeostasis of essential trace elements such as copper and zinc in the body [53]. Cd exposure stimulates the synthesis of hepatic Mts, which bind with Cd^{2+} to form Cd–MT complexes to reduce the damage caused by free Cd^{2+} [53]. Previous studies have indicated that combined exposure to Se and Cd results in the formation of Cd–Se complexes or Cd–Se protein complexes [54,55]. Therefore, the presence of endogenous Se in *Cv2* may have led to the formation of inert complexes with Cd^{2+}, reducing the need for Mts in the organism.

Furthermore, selenoproteins partly participated in alleviating the negative effects of the HFD and Cd exposure. SELENOP is essential in maintaining the homeostasis of selenoproteins and is also associated with lipid metabolism [56]. Elevated circulating levels of SELENOP have been observed in obese individuals [57], and a deficiency in Selenof [58],

Selenom [59], Selenos [60], Selenot [61], or Selenov [62] has been shown to lead to lipid metabolic disorder in established mouse models and usually exacerbates HFD-induced lipid accumulation in the body. At the same dietary Se level, the *Cv1*D and *Cv1*HFD groups had no differences in the mRNA abundance of the selenogenome, regardless of the dietary fat content. The supplementation of *Cv2* not only significantly increased the Se concentrations in the livers of the *Cv2*HFD group but also differentially regulated the mRNA expression levels of some selenoproteins. Previous studies have indicated that selenoproteins, particularly some endoplasmic reticulum-resident selenoproteins, play crucial roles in mediating Se's antagonism against Cd-induced hepatic toxicity [63]. Interestingly, we observed that the protein abundance of some selenoproteins in the liver was not consistent with their corresponding mRNA expression. This may be caused by Cd in *Cv2* inhibiting the biosynthesis of selenoproteins and Se metabolites to weaken the beneficial effects of Se on the organism [63]. In addition, the suppression of selenoprotein synthesis by Cd may also be due to the formation of the above-mentioned Cd–Se complex [63,64]. Although the specific selenoproteins involved and their respective abilities to bind Cd are not yet clear, the significantly changed protein levels of Dio3, Selenoh, and Selenoi in the *Cv2*HFD group suggest that these selenoproteins may have specific roles in mediating Se's effect in the interaction of the HFD and Cd.

Lastly, it should be noted that our study has certain limitations: although the Se content was higher and the Cd content was lower in *Cv2*HFD in our study than in previous studies [8,9], we were unable to evaluate in detail the impact of the interaction between Se and Cd on HFD-induced health damage due to a shortage of *Cv* with high Se as in *Cv2*, low Cd as in *Cv1*, low Se as in *Cv1*, or high Cd as in *Cv2* without exogenous element supplementation. Furthermore, previous studies have reported that, in Se–Cd-coenriched plants, Se could alter the forms and toxicity of Cd to the body [13,14,64]. However, we did not identify the forms of Cd present in *Cv2* or their different impacts on health. Therefore, future studies need to illuminate the interaction between Se and Cd in the soil–plant–organism system in Se–Cd-rich areas. It would also be worthwhile to further investigate the utilization and safety of Se, changes in Cd toxicity in Se–Cd-coenriched agricultural products, and the impact of the interaction between Se, Cd, and the HFD on overall health.

5. Conclusions

In summary, our study suggests that, in the presence of Cd accumulation, *Cv2* still demonstrates effects in terms of alleviating the elevated levels of serum TC and TG, as well as liver lipid deposition, histological damage, and oxidative stress, in HFD mice. The observed beneficial effects of *Cv2* on HFD-induced metabolic disorder were probably associated with its unique Se speciation to antagonize the combined exposure to the HFD and Cd via its regulation of the expression of specific lipid metabolic genes and selenoproteins. However, the current study suggests that, when considering the consumption of Se-enriched agricultural products as a means of Se supplementation, it is necessary to evaluate the potential toxicity caused by the coaccumulation of Cd. Further research is still needed to explore the interaction of Se, Cd, and the HFD and its effects on health to provide a better reference for the development of Se supplements and Se-enriched agricultural products originating from naturally Se–Cd-rich areas.

Supplementary Materials: The following supporting information can be downloaded at https://www.mdpi.com/article/10.3390/nu16183208/s1, Figure S1: Accumulation of copper, iron, and zinc in the livers of adult female mice; Figure S2: Blood glucose changes in OGTT and ITT; Figure S3: The relative mRNA expression of three ER selenoproteins and three non-ER selenoproteins; Table S1: Primer sequences for qPCR; Table S2: Target protein, type, dilution, and source of primary antibodies used for the Western blot analyses.

Author Contributions: Conceptualization, J.-C.Z. and X.G.L.; Methodology, J.Z., Q.L., F.L., P.X., Z.H., A.Y., C.W. and J.J.; Resources, Y.Z., X.C., and L.S.; Formal analysis, J.Z., Q.L., F.L. and P.X.; Visualization, J.Z., Q.L., F.L. and P.X.; Supervision, J.-C.Z. and X.G.L.; Project administration, J.-C.Z.

and X.G.L.; Writing—original draft preparation, J.Z.; Writing—review and editing, Q.L., F.L., P.X., Z.H., A.Y., Z.S., X.G.L. and J.-C.Z.; Funding acquisition, J.-C.Z. All authors have read and agreed to the published version of the manuscript.

Funding: This work was supported by the Science, Technology and Innovation Commission of Shenzhen Municipality, China (GJHZ20240218114600001) and the National Natural Science Foundation of China (81973038) to J.C.Z.

Institutional Review Board Statement: The experiments were approved by the Animal Care and Use Committee of the Institute of Sun Yat-sen University (SYSU-IACUC-2019-B505, 5 March 2019).

Informed Consent Statement: Not applicable.

Data Availability Statement: Data are contained within the article.

Acknowledgments: We would like to acknowledge Zhoutian Wang, Aiping Liu, and Minning Chen for their technical support in the animal experiments.

Conflicts of Interest: The authors declare no conflicts of interest.

References

1. Ramírez-Acosta, S.; Huertas-Abril, P.V.; Selma-Royo, M.; Prieto-Álamo, M.J.; Collado, M.C.; Abril, N.; García-Barrera, T. The role of selenium in shaping mice brain metabolome and selenoproteome through the gut-brain axis by combining metabolomics, metallomics, gene expression, and amplicon sequencing. *J. Nutr. Biochem.* **2023**, *117*, 109323. [CrossRef] [PubMed]
2. Hadrup, N.; Ravn-Haren, G. Toxicity of repeated oral intake of organic selenium, inorganic selenium, and selenium nanoparticles: A review. *J. Trace Elem. Med. Biol. Organ Soc. Miner. Trace Elem. (GMS)* **2023**, *79*, 127235. [CrossRef] [PubMed]
3. Somagattu, P.; Chinnannan, K.; Yammanuru, H.; Reddy, U.K.; Nimmakayala, P. Selenium dynamics in plants: Uptake, transport, toxicity, and sustainable management strategies. *Sci. Total Environ.* **2024**, *949*, 175033. [CrossRef] [PubMed]
4. Liu, X.M.; Yuan, Z.G.; Rao, S.; Zhang, W.W.; Ye, J.B.; Cheng, S.Y.; Xu, F. Identification, characterization, and expression analysis of WRKY transcription factors in *Cardamine violifolia* reveal the key genes involved in regulating selenium accumulation. *BMC Plant Biol.* **2024**, *24*, 860. [CrossRef]
5. Cui, L.; Zhao, J.; Chen, J.; Zhang, W.; Gao, Y.; Li, B.; Li, Y.-F. Translocation and transformation of selenium in hyperaccumulator plant *Cardamine enshiensis* from Enshi, Hubei, China. *Plant Soil* **2018**, *425*, 577–588. [CrossRef]
6. Guo, R.; Ren, R.; Wang, L.; Zhi, Q.; Yu, T.; Hou, Q.; Yang, Z. Using machine learning to predict selenium and cadmium contents in rice grains from black shale-distributed farmland area. *Sci. Total Environ.* **2024**, *912*, 168802. [CrossRef]
7. Feng, R.; Wei, C.; Tu, S.; Ding, Y.; Song, Z. A dual role of Se on Cd toxicity: Evidences from the uptake of Cd and some essential elements and the growth responses in paddy rice. *Biol. Trace Elem. Res.* **2013**, *151*, 113–121. [CrossRef]
8. Zhang, L.; Shi, W.Y.; Xu, J.Y.; Liu, Y.; Wang, S.J.; Zheng, J.Y.; Li, Y.H.; Yuan, L.X.; Qin, L.Q. Protective effects and mechanism of chemical- and plant-based selenocystine against cadmium-induced liver damage. *J. Hazard. Mater.* **2024**, *468*, 133812. [CrossRef]
9. Zhang, L.; Shi, W.Y.; Zhang, L.L.; Sha, Y.; Xu, J.Y.; Shen, L.C.; Li, Y.H.; Yuan, L.X.; Qin, L.Q. Effects of selenium-cadmium co-enriched *Cardamine hupingshanensis* on bone damage in mice. *Ecotoxicol. Environ. Saf.* **2024**, *272*, 116101. [CrossRef]
10. Zhu, H.; Tang, X.; Gu, C.; Chen, R.; Liu, Y.; Chu, H.; Zhang, Z. Assessment of human exposure to cadmium and its nephrotoxicity in the Chinese population. *Sci. Total Environ.* **2024**, *918*, 170488. [CrossRef]
11. Baba, H.; Tsuneyama, K.; Yazaki, M.; Nagata, K.; Minamisaka, T.; Tsuda, T.; Nomoto, K.; Hayashi, S.; Miwa, S.; Nakajima, T.; et al. The liver in itai-itai disease (chronic cadmium poisoning): Pathological features and metallothionein expression. *Mod. Pathol.* **2013**, *26*, 1228–1234. [CrossRef] [PubMed]
12. Huang, N.; Wang, B.; Liu, S.; Wang, K.; Wang, R.; Liu, F.; Chen, C. Cadmium exposure in infants and children: Toxicity, health effects, dietary risk assessment and mitigation strategies. *Crit. Rev. Food Sci. Nutr.* **2024**, 1–23. [CrossRef] [PubMed]
13. Ismael, M.A.; Elyamine, A.M.; Moussa, M.G.; Cai, M.; Zhao, X.; Hu, C. Cadmium in plants: Uptake, toxicity, and its interactions with selenium fertilizers. *Metallomics* **2019**, *11*, 255–277. [CrossRef] [PubMed]
14. Yang, R.; He, Y.; Luo, L.; Zhu, M.; Zan, S.; Guo, F.; Wang, B.; Yang, B. The interaction between selenium and cadmium in the soil-rice-human continuum in an area with high geological background of selenium and cadmium. *Ecotoxicol. Environ. Saf.* **2021**, *222*, 112516. [CrossRef] [PubMed]
15. Chen, J.; He, W.; Zhu, X.; Yang, S.; Yu, T.; Ma, W. Epidemiological study of kidney health in an area with high levels of soil cadmium and selenium: Does selenium protect against cadmium-induced kidney injury? *Sci. Total Environ.* **2020**, *698*, 134106. [CrossRef]
16. Boutari, C.; Mantzoros, C.S. A 2022 update on the epidemiology of obesity and a call to action: As its twin COVID-19 pandemic appears to be receding, the obesity and dysmetabolism pandemic continues to rage on. *Metab. Clin. Exp.* **2022**, *133*, 155217. [CrossRef]
17. Global burden of 369 diseases and injuries in 204 countries and territories, 1990–2019: A systematic analysis for the Global Burden of Disease Study 2019. *Lancet* **2020**, *396*, 1204–1222. [CrossRef]
18. Loomba, R.; Friedman, S.L.; Shulman, G.I. Mechanisms and disease consequences of nonalcoholic fatty liver disease. *Cell* **2021**, *184*, 2537–2564. [CrossRef]

19. Świątkiewicz, I.; Wróblewski, M.; Nuszkiewicz, J.; Sutkowy, P.; Wróblewska, J.; Woźniak, A. The role of oxidative stress enhanced by adiposity in cardiometabolic diseases. *Int. J. Mol. Sci.* **2023**, *24*, 6382. [CrossRef]
20. Wang, P.; Lu, Z.; He, M.; Shi, B.; Lei, X.; Shan, A. The effects of endoplasmic-reticulum-resident selenoproteins in a nonalcoholic fatty liver disease pig model induced by a high-fat diet. *Nutrients* **2020**, *12*, 692. [CrossRef]
21. Zhao, Z.; Kim, J.; Lei, X.G. High Dietary Fat and Selenium Concentrations Exert Tissue- and Glutathione Peroxidase 1-Dependent Impacts on Lipid Metabolism of Young-Adult Mice. *J. Nutr.* **2020**, *150*, 1738–1748. [CrossRef] [PubMed]
22. Wang, X.; Wu, B.; Sun, G.; Gao, J.; Huang, T.; Liu, J.; Zhou, Q.; He, X.; Zhang, S.; Wang, C.Y.; et al. Dietary selenomethionine attenuates obesity by enhancing beiging process in white adipose tissue. *J. Nutr. Biochem.* **2023**, *113*, 109230. [CrossRef] [PubMed]
23. Yu, T.; Guo, J.; Zhu, S.; Li, M.; Zhu, Z.; Cheng, S.; Wang, S.; Sun, Y.; Cong, X. Protective effects of selenium-enriched peptides from *Cardamine violifolia* against high-fat diet induced obesity and its associated metabolic disorders in mice. *RSC Adv.* **2020**, *10*, 31411–31424. [CrossRef] [PubMed]
24. Zhou, W.; Young, J.L.; Men, H.; Zhang, H.; Yu, H.; Lin, Q.; Xu, H.; Xu, J.; Tan, Y.; Zheng, Y.; et al. Sex differences in the effects of whole-life, low-dose cadmium exposure on postweaning high-fat diet-induced cardiac pathogeneses. *Sci. Total Environ.* **2022**, *809*, 152176. [CrossRef]
25. Young, J.L.; Yan, X.; Xu, J.; Yin, X.; Zhang, X.; Arteel, G.E.; Barnes, G.N.; States, J.C.; Watson, W.H.; Kong, M.; et al. Cadmium and High-Fat Diet Disrupt Renal, Cardiac and Hepatic Essential Metals. *Sci. Rep.* **2019**, *9*, 14675. [CrossRef]
26. Liu, T.; Liang, X.; Lei, C.; Huang, Q.; Song, W.; Fang, R.; Li, C.; Li, X.; Mo, H.; Sun, N.; et al. High-Fat Diet Affects Heavy Metal Accumulation and Toxicity to Mice Liver and Kidney Probably via Gut Microbiota. *Front. Microbiol.* **2020**, *11*, 1604. [CrossRef]
27. Wang, J.; Song, Y.; Elsherif, L.; Song, Z.; Zhou, G.; Prabhu, S.D.; Saari, J.T.; Cai, L. Cardiac metallothionein induction plays the major role in the prevention of diabetic cardiomyopathy by zinc supplementation. *Circulation* **2006**, *113*, 544–554. [CrossRef]
28. Zhang, X.; Xia, H.; Wang, J.; Leng, R.; Zhou, X.; Gao, Q.; He, K.; Liu, D.; Huang, B. Effect of selenium-enriched kiwifruit on body fat reduction and liver protection in hyperlipidaemic mice. *Food Funct.* **2021**, *12*, 2044–2057. [CrossRef]
29. Shang, L.; Li, F.; Zhu, J.; Sun, C.; Wang, Y. Selenium-enriched and ordinary black teas regulate the metabolism of glucose and lipid and intestinal flora of hyperglycemic mice. *Plant Foods Hum. Nutr.* **2023**, *78*, 61–67. [CrossRef]
30. Gu, J.; Kong, A.; Guo, C.; Liu, J.; Li, K.; Ren, Z.; Zhou, Y.; Tang, M.; Shi, H. Cadmium perturbed lipid profile and induced liver dysfunction in mice through phosphatidylcholine remodeling and promoting arachidonic acid synthesis and metabolism. *Ecotoxicol. Environ. Saf.* **2022**, *247*, 114254. [CrossRef]
31. Liu, Y.; Kang, W.; Liu, S.; Li, J.; Liu, J.; Chen, X.; Gan, F.; Huang, K. Gut microbiota-bile acid-intestinal Farnesoid X receptor signaling axis orchestrates cadmium-induced liver injury. *Sci. Total Environ.* **2022**, *849*, 157861. [CrossRef] [PubMed]
32. Chen, Z.; Shi, K.; Kuang, W.; Huang, L. Exploration of the optimal strategy for dietary calcium intervention against the toxicity of liver and kidney induced by cadmium in mice: An in vivo diet intervention study. *PLoS ONE* **2021**, *16*, e0250885. [CrossRef] [PubMed]
33. Young, J.L.; Cave, M.C.; Xu, Q.; Kong, M.; Xu, J.; Lin, Q.; Tan, Y.; Cai, L. Whole life exposure to low dose cadmium alters diet-induced NAFLD. *Toxicol. Appl. Pharmacol.* **2022**, *436*, 115855. [CrossRef] [PubMed]
34. Hu, X.; Chandler, J.D.; Fernandes, J.; Orr, M.L.; Hao, L.; Uppal, K.; Neujahr, D.C.; Jones, D.P.; Go, Y.M. Selenium supplementation prevents metabolic and transcriptomic responses to cadmium in mouse lung. *Biochim. Biophys. Acta Gen. Subj.* **2018**, *1862*, 2417–2426. [CrossRef] [PubMed]
35. Zhang, X.; Li, X.; Sheng, Z.; Wang, S.; Li, B.; Tao, S.; Zhang, Z. Effects of combined exposure to cadmium and high-fat diet on bone quality in male mice. *Biol. Trace Elem. Res.* **2020**, *193*, 434–444. [CrossRef]
36. Navarro-Alarcon, M.; Cabrera-Vique, C. Selenium in food and the human body: A review. *Sci. Total Environ.* **2008**, *400*, 115–141. [CrossRef]
37. Genchi, G.; Sinicropi, M.S.; Lauria, G.; Carocci, A.; Catalano, A. The Effects of Cadmium Toxicity. *Int. J. Environ. Res. Public Health* **2020**, *17*, 3782. [CrossRef]
38. Xu, Y.R.; Talukder, M.; Li, C.X.; Zhang, C.; Ge, J.; Li, J.L. Nanoselenium alleviates cadmium-induced cerebral injury via regulating cerebral metal transporters and metal-regulatory transcription factor 1. *J. Agric. Food Chem.* **2023**, *71*, 9896–9907. [CrossRef]
39. Wang, Y.; Hou, J.; Li, X.; Chen, P.; Chen, F.; Pan, Y.; Deng, Z.; Li, J.; Liu, R.; Luo, T. Tyrosol regulates hepatic lipid metabolism in high-fat diet-induced NAFLD mice. *Food Funct.* **2024**, *15*, 3752–3764. [CrossRef]
40. Lv, C.; Liu, X.; Chen, S.; Yi, Y.; Wen, X.; Li, T.; Qin, S. Extract of Gardenia jasminoides Ellis Attenuates High-Fat Diet-Induced Glycolipid Metabolism Disorder in Rats by Targeting Gut Microbiota and TLR4/Myd88/NF-κB Pathway. *Antioxidants* **2024**, *13*, 293. [CrossRef]
41. He, X.; Qi, Z.; Hou, H.; Gao, J.; Zhang, X.X. Effects of chronic cadmium exposure at food limitation-relevant levels on energy metabolism in mice. *J. Hazard. Mater.* **2020**, *388*, 121791. [CrossRef] [PubMed]
42. Song, Y.; Zhang, J.; Li, Y.; Wang, Y.; Wan, Y. Potential Protective Effect of Selenium-Enriched Lactobacillus plantarum on Cadmium-Induced Liver Injury in Mice. *J. Microbiol. Biotechnol.* **2024**, *34*, 1328–1339. [CrossRef] [PubMed]
43. Wan, X.M.; Chen, J.; Wang, M.; Zheng, C.; Zhou, X.L. Puerarin attenuates cadmium-induced hepatic lipid metabolism disorder by inhibiting oxidative stress and inflammation in mice. *J. Inorg. Biochem.* **2021**, *222*, 111521. [CrossRef] [PubMed]
44. Zhou, Y.; Chen, X.; Su, T.; Yuan, M.; Sun, X. Kiwifruit Peel Extract Improves the Alterations in Lipid Metabolism in High-fat Diet-fed Model Rats. *Plant Foods Hum. Nutr.* **2024**, *79*, 113–119. [CrossRef] [PubMed]

45. Luo, J.; Yang, H.; Song, B.L. Mechanisms and regulation of cholesterol homeostasis. *Nat. Rev. Mol. Cell Biol.* **2020**, *21*, 225–245. [CrossRef]
46. Rezaei, F.; Farhat, D.; Gursu, G.; Samnani, S.; Lee, J.Y. Snapshots of ABCG1 and ABCG5/G8: A Sterol's Journey to Cross the Cellular Membranes. *Int. J. Mol. Sci.* **2022**, *24*, 484. [CrossRef]
47. Funes, A.K.; Avena, V.; Boarelli, P.V.; Monclus, M.A.; Zoppino, D.F.; Saez-Lancellotti, T.E.; Fornes, M.W. Cholesterol dynamics in rabbit liver: High-fat diet, olive oil, and synergistic dietary effects. *Biochem. Biophys. Res. Commun.* **2024**, *733*, 150675. [CrossRef]
48. Ogushi, S.; Kimura, T. The difference in zinc concentrations required for induction among metallothionein isoforms can be explained by the different MTF1 affinities to MREs in its promoter. *Int. J. Mol. Sci.* **2023**, *24*, 283. [CrossRef]
49. Nordberg, M.; Nordberg, G.F. Metallothionein and Cadmium Toxicology-Historical Review and Commentary. *Biomolecules* **2022**, *12*, 360. [CrossRef]
50. Lindeque, J.Z.; Jansen van Rensburg, P.J.; Louw, R.; van der Westhuizen, F.H.; Florit, S.; Ramírez, L.; Giralt, M.; Hidalgo, J. Obesity and metabolomics: Metallothioneins protect against high-fat diet-induced consequences in metallothionein knockout mice. *Omics A J. Integr. Biol.* **2015**, *19*, 92–103. [CrossRef]
51. Sato, M.; Kawakami, T.; Kondoh, M.; Takiguchi, M.; Kadota, Y.; Himeno, S.; Suzuki, S. Development of high-fat-diet-induced obesity in female metallothionein-null mice. *FASEB J. Off. Publ. Fed. Am. Soc. Exp. Biol.* **2010**, *24*, 2375–2384. [CrossRef] [PubMed]
52. Banni, M.; Messaoudi, I.; Said, L.; El Heni, J.; Kerkeni, A.; Said, K. Metallothionein gene expression in liver of rats exposed to cadmium and supplemented with zinc and selenium. *Arch. Environ. Contam. Toxicol.* **2010**, *59*, 513–519. [CrossRef] [PubMed]
53. Cirovic, A.; Cirovic, A.; Yimthiang, S.; Vesey, D.A.; Satarug, S. Modulation of Adverse Health Effects of Environmental Cadmium Exposure by Zinc and Its Transporters. *Biomolecules* **2024**, *14*, 650. [CrossRef] [PubMed]
54. Gasiewicz, T.A.; Smith, J.C. Properties of the cadmium and selenium complex formed in rat plasma in vivo and in vitro. *Chem.-Biol. Interact.* **1978**, *23*, 171–183. [CrossRef] [PubMed]
55. Gasiewicz, T.A.; Smith, J.C. Interaction between cadmium and selenium in rat plasma. *Environ. Health Perspect.* **1978**, *25*, 133–136. [CrossRef] [PubMed]
56. Yu, R.; Wang, Z.; Ma, M.; Xu, P.; Liu, L.; Tinkov, A.A.; Lei, X.G.; Zhou, J.C. Associations between Circulating SELENOP Level and Disorders of Glucose and Lipid Metabolism: A Meta-Analysis. *Antioxidants* **2022**, *11*, 1263. [CrossRef]
57. Chen, M.; Liu, B.; Wilkinson, D.; Hutchison, A.T.; Thompson, C.H.; Wittert, G.A.; Heilbronn, L.K. Selenoprotein P is elevated in individuals with obesity, but is not independently associated with insulin resistance. *Obes. Res. Clin. Pract.* **2017**, *11*, 227–232. [CrossRef]
58. Zheng, X.; Ren, B.; Li, X.; Yan, H.; Xie, Q.; Liu, H.; Zhou, J.; Tian, J.; Huang, K. Selenoprotein F knockout leads to glucose and lipid metabolism disorders in mice. *J. Biol. Inorg. Chem.* **2020**, *25*, 1009–1022. [CrossRef]
59. Cai, J.; Huang, J.; Yang, J.; Chen, X.; Zhang, H.; Zhu, Y.; Liu, Q.; Zhang, Z. The protective effect of selenoprotein M on non-alcoholic fatty liver disease: The role of the AMPKα1–MFN2 pathway and Parkin mitophagy. *Cell. Mol. Life Sci. CMLS* **2022**, *79*, 354. [CrossRef]
60. Qiao, L.; Men, L.; Yu, S.; Yao, J.; Li, Y.; Wang, M.; Yu, Y.; Wang, N.; Ran, L.; Wu, Y.; et al. Hepatic deficiency of selenoprotein S exacerbates hepatic steatosis and insulin resistance. *Cell Death Dis.* **2022**, *13*, 275. [CrossRef]
61. Li, K.; Feng, T.; Liu, L.; Liu, H.; Huang, K.; Zhou, J. Hepatic proteomic analysis of selenoprotein T knockout mice by TMT: Implications for the role of selenoprotein T in glucose and lipid metabolism. *Int. J. Mol. Sci.* **2021**, *22*, 8515. [CrossRef] [PubMed]
62. Chen, L.-L.; Huang, J.-Q.; Wu, Y.-Y.; Chen, L.-B.; Li, S.-P.; Zhang, X.; Wu, S.; Ren, F.-Z.; Lei, X.-G. Loss of Selenov predisposes mice to extra fat accumulation and attenuated energy expenditure. *Redox Biol.* **2021**, *45*, 102048. [CrossRef] [PubMed]
63. Ramírez-Acosta, S.; Uhlírová, R.; Navarro, F.; Gómez-Ariza, J.L.; García-Barrera, T. Antagonistic interaction of selenium and cadmium in human hepatic cells through selenoproteins. *Front. Chem.* **2022**, *10*, 891933. [CrossRef] [PubMed]
64. Zhang, L.; Yang, F.; Li, Y.; Cao, H.; Huang, A.; Zhuang, Y.; Zhang, C.; Hu, G.; Mao, Y.; Luo, J.; et al. The protection of selenium against cadmium-induced mitophagy via modulating nuclear xenobiotic receptors response and oxidative stress in the liver of rabbits. *Environ. Pollut.* **2021**, *285*, 117301. [CrossRef] [PubMed]

nutrients

MDPI

Review

Selenium and Skeletal Muscle Health in Sports Nutrition

Qi Wang [1], Jiaqiang Huang [2,3], Kongdi Zhu [2,3,*] and Wei Zuo [1,*]

1 Institute of Artificial Intelligence in Sports, Capital University of Physical Education and Sports, Beijing 100083, China; 00020240005@cupes.edu.cn
2 Beijing Advanced Innovation Center for Food Nutrition and Human Health, Department of Nutrition and Health, China Agricultural University, Beijing 100083, China; jqhuang@cau.edu.cn
3 Key Laboratory of Precision Nutrition and Food Quality, Ministry of Education, Department of Nutrition and Health, China Agricultural University, Beijing 100083, China
* Correspondence: zkd15938702692@163.com (K.Z.); zuowei@cupes.edu.cn (W.Z.)

Abstract: Selenium is a trace element of fundamental importance to human health. In recent years, an increasing number of studies have been carried out in the field of skeletal muscle health and sports nutrition. Selenium functions in the human body through selenoproteins. Selenoproteins play an important role in maintaining skeletal muscle function by delaying exercise fatigue and muscle aging. They mainly regulate skeletal muscle by anti-oxidation, regulating signal pathways, and affecting protein metabolism. In this paper, we summarize the latest advancements in research regarding selenium and its impact on skeletal muscle health, along with its applications in sports nutrition.

Keywords: selenium; selenoprotein; skeletal muscle health

1. Introduction

Selenium functions in the body mainly through selenoproteins. Selenoproteins are a special protein family containing the 21st amino acid (selenocysteine, Sec) [1,2]. Sec is translated by the UGA stop codon and inserted into the protein. In eukaryotes, the SEC-insertion sequence (SECIS) element located in the 3′-untranslated region (3′UTR) of selenoprotein mRNA distinguishes between the UGA codon used to translate Sec and the UGA stop codon and recognizes the binding of SECIS binding protein (SBP2) to it [3,4]. Thus, selenoprotein synthesis can be completed. So far, 25 selenium proteins have been found in humans [5]. These selenoproteins have a variety of biological functions—including regulation of thyroid hormone metabolism, intracellular and extracellular antioxidation, reverse transport of proteins from endoplasmic reticulum to cytoplasm, etc.—which play an important role in maintaining the homeostasis of cells and tissues and the health of the body [6]. Se deficiency in individuals may cause a variety of diseases, such as tissue oxidative stress, white muscle disease, and even cancer.

Skeletal muscle is a main target organ for tissue damage caused by Se deficiency. The skeletal muscle tissue will be dysfunctional when organisms are deficient in selenium. Se deficiency may eventually lead to impaired muscle contraction, muscle necrosis, and atrophy, due to vascular injury, degeneration, and extensive calcification [7,8]. Selenium deficiency affects the recovery of muscle atrophy and directly causes metabolic disorder in skeletal muscle, which, in turn, affects the normal physiological function of skeletal muscle [9]. Skeletal muscle represents the most massive tissue in the body in adult mammals [10]. Following injury, skeletal muscle displays a powerful regenerative capacity that is attributed to the ordered regulation of a cascade of events initiated by satellite cells

(SCs). Skeletal muscle is indispensable for critical physiological functions, including locomotion, postural stabilization, respiratory mechanics, and thermoregulation. This tissue predominantly consists of multinucleated myofibers formed through mitotic fusion during development. The homeostatic maintenance and repair of muscle tissue are facilitated by resident SCs, which reside in a quiescent state between the basal lamina and sarcolemma of myofibers. Under physiological conditions, SCs remain primed for activation in response to mechanical injury or exogenous growth signals, initiating myogenic differentiation and regeneration processes to preserve tissue integrity [11]. Emerging evidence highlights the critical importance of selenium and selenoproteins in skeletal muscle biology, particularly their roles in reducing exercise-induced fatigue, improving post-exercise recovery, and combating age-related muscle decline. However, the comprehensive mechanisms through which Se and selenoproteins maintain skeletal muscle health remain to be fully elucidated. This review systematically consolidates current knowledge regarding selenium's biological mechanisms, focusing on three key aspects, i.e., (1) antioxidant regulation, (2) mitochondrial function modulation, and (3) protein metabolism regulation, while discussing their practical applications for enhancing athletic performance and maintaining muscle health.

2. Selenoproteins in Skeletal Muscle Biology

Se mediates its physiological roles in mammals predominantly through selenoproteins. Of the 25 selenoproteins identified thus far in mammals, two (GPX4 and TXNRD2) are classified as mitochondrial selenoproteins, while seven others (DIO2, SELENOF, SELENOK, SELENOS, SELENOM, SELENON, and SELENOT) are localized in the endoplasmic reticulum [5]. These selenoproteins have the ability to regulate mitochondrial and endoplasmic reticulum (ER) homeostasis. Previous studies have focused on the function of individual selenium proteins. Jing et al. showed that the biological function of selenoproteins is not a single one, but a synergistic function of multiple selenoproteins [12]. We describe the mechanisms by which selenium supplementation exerts its effects in muscle cells in the form of selenoproteins to promote exercise fitness in Figure 1.

2.1. SELENOW

Selenoprotein W (SELENOW) is a skeletal muscle-enriched selenoprotein with a thioredoxin-like fold; it belongs to the Rdx family. It was the first selenoprotein described to be linked to white muscle disease in lambs [13]. Numerous studies have demonstrated that SELENOW can function in redox regulation [14,15], cell cycle progression [16], and myogenic differentiation [17,18], which are related to muscle growth and development. It also plays a pivotal role in calcium homeostasis and proteostasis. During selenium deficiency, downregulation of SELENOW disrupts the STIM1/TRPC1-mediated calcium influx, leading to impaired myoblast fusion and muscle regeneration. In dexamethasone-induced atrophy models, SELENOW knockout mice exhibited exacerbated muscle loss via suppression of RAC1-mTOR signaling and activation of ubiquitin ligases (MuRF1/Atrogin-1) [19]. Clinically, SELENOW expression is positively correlated with grip strength in elderly populations, suggesting its potential as a biomarker for sarcopenia [20].

SELENOW also plays a pivotal role in redox regulation through its interaction with GSH [19]. Mechanistically, under oxidative stress, glutathione S-transferase Pi (GSTP1) catalyzes the S-glutathionylation of murine SELENOW at cysteine residue 33 (Cys33). This post-translational modification prevents the formation of a second disulfide bond within SELENOW, thereby enhancing its capacity to mitigate oxidative damage and maintain cellular viability [15].

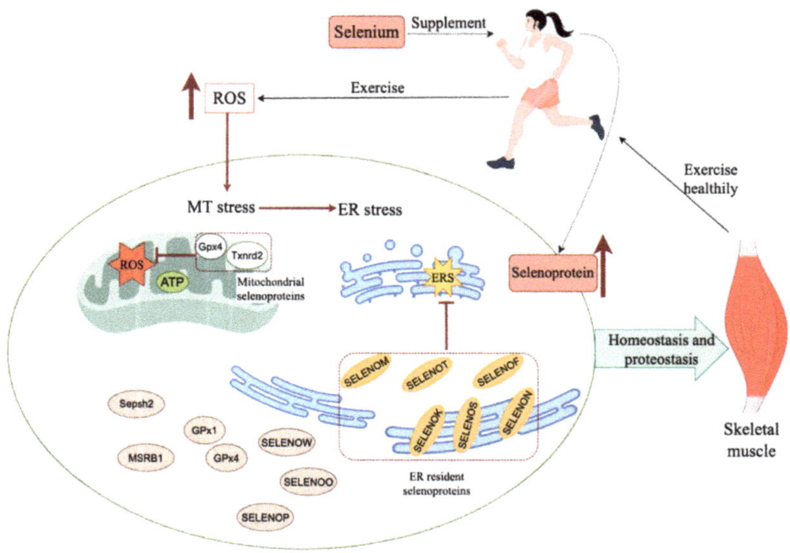

Figure 1. Synergistic effects of selenoprotein networks in skeletal muscle. Several key selenoproteins collaborate to eliminate excess ROS, alleviate mitochondrial and ER stress, and restore cellular homeostasis disrupted by oxidative stress induced by excessive exercise. Moderate selenium supplementation helps maintain skeletal muscle homeostasis and protease balance, thereby enhancing exercise performance and fitness. ER: endoplasmic reticulum; ERS: endoplasmic reticulum stress; ROS: reactive oxygen species; MT:mitochondria.The red up thick arrow in the figure indicates the increase in number. The figure was created with https://www.figdraw.com/ (accessed on 10 May 2025).

2.2. SELENON

Selenoprotein N (SELENON) is an ER protein whose loss of function leads to human SELENON-related myopathies [21]. It has a thioredoxin reductase-like domain on the ER side of its sequence and regulates ER calcium levels by means of the redox regulating SERCA2 pump [22]. SELENON directly interacts with ryanodine receptors (RyRs), constituting critical components of calcium release channels which serve as molecular regulators of endoplasmic reticulum calcium homeostasis and redox equilibrium [23–25]. SELENON is a selenoprotein that is widely recognized to play an important role in skeletal muscle diseases. In the presence of selenium deficiency, decreased SELENON content leads to decreased calcium release from the sarcoplasmic reticulum and increased production of tonic contraction-associated ROS, directly leading to skeletal muscle pain, fatigue, and proximal weakness that contribute to polyaxial disease, congenital muscular dystrophy, and sarcopenia during aging, changes that can be alleviated by selenium, and sarcopenia during aging, changes that can be alleviated by selenium supplementation [26,27].

2.3. SELENOK

Selenoprotein K (SELENOK) is also an ER protein. It is abundantly expressed in muscle tissue and has functions such as the degradation of ER-related proteins, anti-oxidation, regulation of Ca^{2+} flux in the ER, and participation in immune response. Previous studies have shown that SELENOK knockdown can cause an imbalance in calcium homeostasis and glucose metabolism in chick embryo myoblasts, as well as impairing muscle development. Studies have shown that SELENOK silencing impairs skeletal muscle repair and inhibits myogenic differentiation of satellite cells. SELENOK plays a key role in regulating the homeostasis of anti-oxidation and ER stress in myoblasts, as well as the level of apoptosis and autophagy. Therefore, SELENOK is involved in the mechanism of satellite cell-led skeletal muscle regeneration. SELENOK binds to a variety of chaperones (p97, SELENOS, Derlin1) on the ER and regulates the intensity of UPR response by promoting ERAD to alleviate ER stress. SELENOK can regulate ER stress by promoting ERAD during skeletal muscle regeneration and regulate antioxidant signaling in an ER stress-dependent manner during myoblast differentiation. Selenoprotein K pro-tects skeletal muscle from damage and is required for SC-mediated myogenic differen-tiation [28,29].

2.4. SELENOS

Selenoprotein S (SELENOS), highly expressed in skeletal muscle, is a transmembrane selenoprotein that resides in the ER and has a C-terminal selenocysteine residue with antioxidant properties and the ability to confer protection against ER stress [30]. In vitro studies have shown that decreased expression of SELENOS (SELENOS) increases oxidative stress and ER stress in various mammalian cell lines [31–33]. Studies have found that SEPS1 has a protective and anti-inflammatory effect in vivo in a lipopolysaccharide (LPS)-induced sepsis mouse model [34]. Genetic polymorphisms of SELENOS are associated with elevated proinflammatory cytokines, and SELENOS has a protective effect against inflammatory stress in vitro. SELENOS polymorphisms can cause congenital muscular dystrophy [35]. Recent studies have identified SELENOS as a novel disease-modifying gene in muscular dystrophy and myopathy by investigating whether genetic depletion of SELENOS in mdx-dystrophic mice exacerbates skeletal muscle inflammation and impairs the structure and function of dystrophic hind limb muscles [36].

2.5. GPx

One of the primary antioxidant systems in cells is catalyzed by the selenoenzyme Glutathione peroxidase (GPx) [37]. The main function of the GPx family is to scavenge ROS and protect cell membrane integrity. GPx1 plays a role in anti-oxidation in the cytoplasm and reducing lipid peroxidation after exercise. GPx4, localized in mitochondria, uniquely prevents ferroptosis by reducing lipid hydroperoxides [19]. In endurance athletes, the activity of muscle GPx increases by 65% post-training, protecting mitochondrial membranes from oxidative rupture [38,39]. Conversely, GPx4 inhibition triggers iron-dependent lipid peroxidation, causing necrotic myofiber death in selenium-deficient models [40].

2.6. Txnrd

Thioredoxin reductase (Txnrd) is an oxidoreductase that catalyzes the reduction of oxidized Thioredoxin (Trx) using NADPH [5]. Trx is, in turn, used by some cellular enzymes as a cofactor in dithio-disulfide bond exchange reactions, which are the main intracellular mechanism for maintaining a reducing environment, especially for the maintenance of reduced cysteine groups. Mammals express three Txnrd isoforms: Txnrd1 (cytoplasmic/nuclear; TR1/TrxR1), responsible for reducing cytosolic thioredoxin (Trx1); Txnrd2 (mitochondrial; TR3/TrxR2), which reduces mitochondrial thioredoxin (Trx2); and Txnrd3 (testis-specific; not discussed here). Notably, cardiomyocyte-specific deletion studies revealed that Txnrd2 is indispensable for viability, underscoring its non-redundant role in maintaining mitochondrial redox homeostasis during cardiac development. This tissue-specific essentiality likely stems from the high energetic demands and ROS exposure inherent to myocardial cells, necessitating robust Txnrd2-mediated antioxidant protection within mitochondria. Based on existing studies, research on the mechanism of TXNRD1 function in sport related fields mainly lies in animal and in vitro verification [41–45].

2.7. MsrB1

Methionine r-sulfoxide reductase (MsrB1) is the main mammalian MsrB located in the cytosol and nucleus. MSRB1 was found to control mammalian actin assembly and breakdown. Micals have been the only known partners of MsrB1, and actin is the only target. This suggests that MSRB1 may be involved in skeletal muscle growth regulation [46]. In addition, MSRB1 is involved in the regulation of redox homeostasis and protects proteins from oxidative damage [47].

2.8. Other Selenoproteins

In addition to the selenoproteins described above, there are a number of selenoproteins that may play a role in maintaining muscle health status. Selenoprotein P (SELENOP) is mainly responsible for the transport of Se from plasma to various target organs, thus controlling the expression of all selenoproteins and SEPHS2 and providing systemic antioxidant defense [12]. Selenoprotein O (SELENOO) is the largest mammalian selenoprotein. SELENOO has been shown to engage in redox interactions with unknown proteins via its CXXU motif. Redox regulation of protein function in mitochondria may involve kinase function [1]. As an ER selenoprotein, Selenoprotein F (SELENOF) can be regulated by both ER stress and selenium status. It may have a functional link with endoplasmic reticulum protein folding and secretion processes. Selenoprotein F (SELENOF) interacts with UDP-glucose:glycoprotein glucosyltransferase (UGGT) to participate in ER quality control mechanisms, ensuring proper folding of nascent glycoproteins. Following successful folding, these proteins are packaged into COPII-coated transport vesicles for anterograde trafficking to the Golgi apparatus, where they undergo post-translational modifications prior to secretion via exocytic pathways [48]. SELENOS is a core component of the reverse translocation channel in ER-related protein degradation, which removes misfolded peptide chains and maintains ER homeostasis. Selenoprotein T (SELENOT) is a member of the thioredoxin-like superfamily containing the CXXU redox-active motif. It mainly has the function of maintaining ER redox balance and regulating autophagy and apoptosis. SELENOT can alleviate ER stress and protect myoblast survival by inhibiting the CHOP/ATF4 pathway. SELENOT knockout exacerbates skeletal muscle aplasia [8]. SELENOK, SELENOT, and SELENOM control ER homeostasis by scavenging excess ROS and inhibiting apoptosis [49–52]. Taking the above analyses together, a summary of the functions of skeletal muscle-associated seloproteins is presented in Table 1. The occurrence of muscle-related diseases is not only related to a single protein but may be caused by multiple proteins together. However, current research is limited, and more in-depth molecular mechanism studies are needed to explore the connection between selenoproteins and muscle-related diseases.

Table 1. Functional summary of skeletal muscle-related selenoproteins.

Selenoprotein	Main Function	Regulatory Pathways/Molecular Mechanisms	Pathological Association	Subcellular Localization	References
SELENOW	Regulates calcium homeostasis, inhibits ubiquitin-proteasome degradation, and promotes muscle tube fusion Protects proliferating myoblasts from the influence of oxidative stress	RAC1-mTOR	Selenium deficiency myopathy and muscular dystrophy	Cytoplasmic	[19,27]

Table 1. *Cont.*

Selenoprotein	Main Function	Regulatory Pathways/Molecular Mechanisms	Pathological Association	Subcellular Localization	References
SELENOT	Maintains the redox balance of ER, inhibits apoptosis and autophagy	CHOP/ATF/SERCA2/ NRF1/PGC-1α PACAP	Muscle aplasia, sports injuries	ER	[53–57]
SELENON	ER redox and calcium homeostasis	RyR1/SERCA	Congenital myopathy (multiple mi-croaxonopathy)	ER	[21,26,27, 58–60]
SELENOK	Participates in repair after skeletal muscle injury	Promote satellite cells-mediated myogenic differentiation; Prevents intracellular antioxidant dysfunction, apoptosis and autophagy by regulating the level of ER stress	Inhibition of skeletal muscle regeneration after injury	ER, plasma membrane	[10]
SELENOP	Selenium transporters maintain systemic selenium homeostasis and enhance antioxidant defense	ApoER2/LRP1 receptor-mediated selenium uptake	Selenium deficiency leads to muscle atrophy and age-related muscle loss	Secreted, cytoplasmic	[12,61,62]
SELENOS	Regulates endoplasmic reticulum-associated degradation (ERAD) to improve insulin sensitivity	SEL1L-HRD1 compound	Skeletal muscle injury and growth retardation due to ER stress	ER	[12,63–65]
GPx1	Removes cytoplasmic hydrogen peroxide (H_2O_2) to protect cell membrane integrity	Nrf2/HO-1; Inhibit oxidative stress and apoptosis; Correct insulin resistance; Regulate fatty acid metabolism;	Oxidative injury after exercise, chronic inflammation	Cytoplasmic	[27,66,67]
GPx4	Specifically inhibits lipid peroxidation and prevents iron death	Lipid peroxidation/ACSL4	Iron death muscle fiber necrosis	Cytoplasmic	[39,68]
SELENOH	Promotes DNA repair and maintains genomic stability	Unknown (possibly related to oxidative damage repair)	DNA damage and muscle fiber degeneration caused by selenium deficiency	Nuclear	[69]
DIO2	Catalyzes the conversion of T4 to T3, regulates thyroid hormone metabolism and energy balance	Thyroid hormone signaling pathway	Metabolic disorders after exercise, muscle fatigue	Membrane-associated	[70,71]

Table 1. *Cont.*

Selenoprotein	Main Function	Regulatory Pathways/Molecular Mechanisms	Pathological Association	Subcellular Localization	References
TXNRD1	Reduction-oxidized thioredoxin, repairs oxidation-damaged protein	Trx/ASK1	Chronic oxidative stress, muscle fibrosis	Cytoplasmic, nuclear	[41–45]
SELENOM	Maintenance of ER homeostasis; regulates glucose metabolism and insulin signal, affects muscle cell energy homeostasis	PI3K-Akt/mTOR	Skeletal muscle injury and growth retardation due to ER stress.	ER	[12,51,72]

3. Mechanisms of Selenium in Muscle Health

Mammalian skeletal muscle accounts for 30–40% of the total body weight and has important physiological functions, including internal organ protection, protein storage, body movement, and thermogenesis [10,73,74]. The physiological hypertrophy of skeletal muscle is characterized by the coordinated accumulation of contractile proteins and limited lipid deposition [75]. Post-exercise oxidative stress (OS) disrupts this process in mammals, resulting in impaired muscle growth through dysregulation of the proteostatic and lipostatic pathways. Mechanistically, OS triggers mitochondrial dysfunction, leading to excessive ROS generation that overwhelms antioxidant defenses. This redox imbalance promotes oxidative modifications of cellular components which concomitantly suppress anabolic signaling while activating catabolic pathways, ultimately driving muscle mass loss [76].

3.1. Antioxidant Defense

Exercise-induced oxidative stress is the result of an increase in free radicals produced by mitochondrial respiration that exceeds antioxidant capacity. Selenium is well-regarded for its role in enhancing muscle function, particularly due to its antioxidant properties. Se supplementation may have significant potential in reducing exercise-induced oxidative stress [77]. The GPx family of selenoproteins serves as a pivotal regulator of ROS-mediated oxidative stress, particularly under conditions of heightened metabolic demand or pathological states such as infection or tissue injury. Through enzymatic reduction of hydroperoxides, GPx isoforms maintain redox homeostasis in skeletal muscle, with their activity being strictly dependent on Se incorporation into the catalytic selenocysteine residue. Notably, mitochondrial GPx4 exhibits compartment-specific functionality by preventing lipid peroxidation within inner mitochondrial membranes, thereby preserving electron transport chain integrity. Collectively, Se-dependent antioxidant systems and mitochondrial bioenergetics constitute critical determinants of skeletal muscle redox balance and metabolic plasticity during stress adaptation [57].

3.2. Mitochondrial Function

Skeletal muscle is the largest energy-consuming tissue in the body, and mitochondria are the main site of aerobic respiration in cells [78], which, besides being the structure of energy production in cells, play an important role in the differentiation, growth, and development and function of various tissues in the body [79,80] Selenium mainly affects the capacity and function of mitochondria, which, in turn, affects muscle health. Dietary selenium supplementation enhances mitochondrial content in skeletal muscle, as evidenced by elevated mitochondrial volume, density, and respiratory complex activity in both in vivo and in vitro models. SELENOH, SELENON, SELENOW, SELENOO, and DIOs show different effects on mitochondrial and/or skeletal muscle function. SELENOH enhances mitochondrial biogenesis, whereas SELENON and SELENOW appear to affect muscle calcium homeostasis and thus mitochondrial function. In addition, the residence of SELENOO within mitochondria contributes to the redox function of Se. Deiodinase regulates thyroid hormone activation, which, in turn, affects muscle cell regeneration, metabolism, and ROS production [57].

There is also research that shows that the depletion of SELENOT leads to the accumulation of mitochondrial superoxide and downregulation of mitochondrial dynamics gene expression, which, in turn, induces disruption of mitochondrial potential and blocks the oxidative phosphorylation process. Mitochondrial ROS overproduction leads to rate limitation of ATP production, accompanied by cell cycle arrest, slow cell proliferation, and increased myocyte apoptosis. The elimination of mitochondrial ROS has been shown to effectively alleviate the above adverse effects and significantly restore the proliferative potential of myoblasts. Therefore, SELENOT acts as a guardian of cellular homeostasis, resisting mitochondrial oxidative stress, protecting ATP production, promoting myoblast proliferation, and inhibiting apoptosis. Despite this, the exact relationship between dietary Se and skeletal muscle mitochondria is currently unknown [8].

3.3. Protein Metabolic Balance

Selenium deficiency disrupts protein turnover by suppressing mTORC1 signaling and activating the ubiquitin-proteasome pathway in skeletal muscle [81]. However, the specific selenoproteins regulating skeletal muscle protein homeostasis remain unclear. The SELENOW-RAC1-mTOR cascade has been proposed as a mechanism coordinating protein synthesis and degradation. In SELENOW-knockout models, reduced EIF4G protein levels and impaired translational activity have been observed. The ubiquitin-proteasome system represents the predominant proteolytic pathway in skeletal muscle [82], driven by the transcription factor FOXO, which upregulates atrophy-associated ubiquitin ligases (Atrogin-1 and MuRF-1) [83]. mTORC2 is essential for AKT-FOXO signaling, while SELENOW modulates both protein synthesis and degradation via the SELENOW-RAC1-mTOR axis, underscoring its critical role in proteostasis [19].

3.4. Calcium Homeostasis and Muscle Contraction

Ca^{2+} is a widespread intracellular signal that can participate in the regulation of a variety of cellular physiological processes. Many effectors downstream of the Ca^{2+} signaling pathway are essential for muscle development, including CAM-dependent kinases and phosphatases, mitogen-activated protein kinases (MAPKs), Ca^{2+} -sensitive transcription factors, and nuclear factor of activated T cells (NFATc) [84]. The role of CAM-dependent phosphatases in mouse myogenesis begins with their function in early skeletal muscle cell differentiation by regulating the expression of transcription factors MEF2, MyoD, and myogenin [85]. In addition to the classic CaM dependent way, other signal cascade may help Ca^{2+} dynamics drive the transduction of skeletal muscle development. Signaling through several elements of the MAPK pathway regulates different steps of myogenesis [86,87]. MAPKs and Ca^{2+} signaling in spinal cord [88] can coordinate the regulation of skeletal muscle development [89].

Ca^{2+} signaling is involved in skeletal muscle development and is directly related to the Ca^{2+} + kinetic patterns of developing muscle cell stored Ca^{2+} access (SOCE), prepared by sensors of internal Ca^{2+} stores, STIM1, SOCE channels Orail, and TRPC channels. STIM1 expression regulates development and peaks in developing mouse muscle [90]. Mice lacking STIM1 die of perinatal skeletal myopathy [91], indicating that STIM1-dependent Ca^{2+} signaling is required for myogenesis. At initiation, TRPC1 expression is also developmentally regulated to differentiate and is required for myoblast migration and fusion into myotubes. SELENOT is involved in the regulation of intracellular calcium concentration in chick embryo myoblasts and significantly affects calcium homeostasis in chick embryo myoblasts. A decrease in SELENOT expression was found to decrease the expression of STIM1 and TRPC1—which are beneficial factors related to muscle development—in calcium channels. Ca^{2+} is an important part of the signal that promotes muscle formation, balance, and regeneration. In particular, changes in Ca^{2+} may directly contribute to muscle satellite cell proliferation or differentiation [9].

4. Selenium Deficiency and Muscle Pathologies

Selenium deficiency impairs maximal contractile strength and isokinetic torque in skeletal muscle, resulting in postural instability and motor dysfunction secondary to myopathic pathologies. This deficiency is further characterized by reduced serum creatine kinase and lactate dehydrogenase activity, correlating with clinical manifestations of skeletal muscle pain and fatigue [92]. Previous studies have reported that Se deficiency is the cause of different forms of cardiac and skeletal muscle disease in humans, termed dystrophic muscular dystrophy [93]. These myopathies are characterized by alterations in cardiac or skeletal muscle fibers, resulting in impaired contraction, muscle atrophy, and varying degrees of limb or trunk stiffness. Keshan disease, a selenium-deficient cardiomyopathy, is characterized by myocardial necrosis, inflammatory infiltration, and calcification. This pathology arises from the synergistic effects of dietary selenium insufficiency and coxsackievirus B3 infection. Selenium deficiency impairs selenoenzyme activity (e.g., GPx), disrupting cardiomyocyte redox homeostasis and potentiating viral DNA oxidative damage. The subsequent accumulation of viral genomic mutations enhances virulence, exacerbating myocardial injury [27].

Sarcopenia is closely related to age-related oxidative stress and the imbalance of protein metabolism. Selenium can delay the progression of muscle atrophy by protecting the function of motor neurons and reducing the degeneration of neuromuscular junction. Clinical studies have shown that people with lower plasma selenium levels are more likely to have decreased hip strength and grip strength [20].

5. Exercise and Skeletal Muscle Adaptation

5.1. Exercise-Induced Increased Selenium Consumption

Intense exercise induces muscle damage, manifesting as delayed-onset muscle soreness and impaired force-generating capacity. This impairment arises from multifactorial mechanisms involving structural disruption of contractile proteins (e.g., myofibrillar Z-disc streaming) and dysregulation of calcium-handling pathways (e.g., sarcoplasmic reticulum Ca^{2+}-ATPase dysfunction). These pathophysiological alterations are mediated by mechanical stress from high-intensity eccentric contractions coupled with the exercise-induced overproduction of ROS, which collectively exacerbate sarcolemmal and organelle membrane permeability [94]. Vigorous exercise increases the production of free radicals or ROS and nitrogen (RONS), which hinder muscle contractile function and lead to muscle fatigue and decreased performance [95]. To combat muscle damage and fatigue and improve performance, athletes often take antioxidant supplements [96]. As an antioxidant, selenium has a strong scavenging capacity for ROS and may exert beneficial effects on exercise performance and exercise recovery in athletic populations. At present, some studies have applied selenium in related studies of exercise training, as shown in Table 2. We found limited human studies showing reduced exertion-related lipid peroxidation in overweight participants with low Se levels [77], whereas several studies have shown no beneficial effects on endurance performance [97–99]. This may be influenced by the form and dose of selenium consumed, as well as the timing of supplementation.

Table 2. Summary of Human Trials on Selenium Supplementation and Exercise Performance.

Forms of Se	Dose	Intervention Duration	Sample Size	Outcome	References
selenomethionine	180 μg/d	10 weeks	24	No effect on the adaptation induced by endurance training	[97]
selenomethionine	240 μg/d	10 weeks	24	Increased the muscle GPx of subjects during acute exercise	[38]
sodium selenite	200 μg/d (Zinc 30 mg/d)	4 weeks	32	Simultaneous and individual supplementation of selenium and zinc had no significant effect on the resting testosterone and lactic acid levels	[98]
sodium selenite	200 μg/d	3 weeks	20	Reduced blood levels of lipid hydroperoxide postexercise in overweight adults	[77]
sodium selenite	17.5 μg/d (Vitamin E 400 IU)	3 weeks	8	Significantly improved endurance exercise performance (VO2max, AT, and endurance performance time), but decreased lactate dehydrogenase (LDH)	[100]
sodium selenite	17.5 μg/d (Vitamin E 400 IU)	3 weeks	9	SOD and GPx were significantly increased and MDA was decreased	[101]
sodium selenite	17.5 μg/d (Vitamin E 400 IU)	3 weeks	10	SOD and GPx were significantly increased, MDA was decreased. Cardiopulmonary endurance (VO2max, AT) was significantly increased	[102]
sodium selenite	17.5 μg/d (Vitamin E 400 IU)	3 weeks	10	SOD and GPX were significantly increased, but MDA was decreased. Vitamin E and selenium significantly reduced blood fatigue factors (NH3, LDH and phosphorus)	[103]
selenium tablets(Not mentioned)	200 μg/d	2 weeks	20	Reduced oxidative stress caused by physical exercise	[104]

5.2. Effect of Selenium Supplementation on Exercise Recovery

Selenium is an essential trace element; deficiencies arising from dietary insufficiency or malabsorption are associated with multiple disorders in humans and livestock, underscoring its critical physiological role. Furthermore, optimal selenium supplementation is hypothesized to confer benefits across diverse aspects of human health. High-intensity exercise elevates ROS generation, correspondingly increasing selenium-dependent antioxidant demands [12]. Dietary antioxidant supplementation represents a therapeutic strategy to mitigate oxidative damage. Se, a core constituent of endogenous antioxidant systems, scavenges excessive ROS and enhances systemic antioxidant capacity through selenoprotein-mediated redox regulation [105,106]. Despite the benefits of selenium supplementation for muscle health, exercise, especially resistance training, remains central to preventing muscle degeneration. High-intensity resistance training combined with selenium supplementation can significantly improve muscle mass and strength, and the effect is better than that of single intervention.

5.3. Dosage and Form of Selenium Supplement

The dose and form of selenium supplements are critical for the effects of selenium. The EFSA has set the dietary reference intake (DRI) of selenium for adults at 70 μg/day and the tolerable upper intake level (UL) at 255 μg/day [107]. The DRI selenium for Chinese residents is 60 μg/day, and the UL is also 400 μg, while the RDI/UL is 55/400 μg per day in US [108]. Selenium levels higher than UL levels result in selenopathy. The main clinical manifestations of this condition are gastrointestinal dysfunction, slow reaction, stiffness of limbs and hair loss. In severe cases, it may cause respiratory failure and death [109]. Therefore, further studies are needed to determine the optimal daily selenium intake for the exercising population and to carry out personalized tailored regimens. Se is supplemented by exogenous intake in humans. It comes from a variety of dietary items including meat, seafood, cereals, dairy products, fruits, vegetables, and some specific Se supplements. Se occurs in many forms in nature. Organic Se (such as selenomethionine and Se yeast) and nano-selenium (SeNPs) have better bioavailability than inorganic Se. Thus, the first two forms of Se should be preferred for the selection of selenium nutritional supplements. In a study of exercising women [110], the consumption of selenium-enriched eggs increased the body's antioxidant capacity, prevented exercise-induced cellular oxidative damage, and delayed the onset of degenerative diseases. Some animal studies have also found that selenium supplementation is beneficial to the improvement of exercise capacity, as mainly reflected in the improvement of antioxidant capacity. The increase in free radical production and lactate levels induced by acute swimming exercise in rats may be offset by sodium selenite supplementation [111,112]. Se supplementation alleviates liver injury induced by exercise fatigue in rats. Se supplementation can also ameliorate oxidative, energetic, metabolic, and endocrine imbalances via modulation of selenoproteins in rat skeletal muscle [113]. Selenium-rich soybean peptides (SePPs) exhibit higher antioxidant and anti-inflammatory activities in vivo than Selenoprotein, SeMet, sodium selenite (Na_2SeO_3), or PPs [114]. (PhSe) 2 was shown to protect against acute physical exercise-induced oxidative damage in mice [115]. SeNPs have also been demonstrated to have tissue antioxidant properties in donkey and grey rabbit, thereby improving exercise fitness [116,117]. However, the optimal timing, dose, and speciation of Se supplementation require further investigation.

6. Clinical Implications and Future Directions

6.1. Intervention Strategies Targeting Selenoproteins

SELENOP is of significant interest due to its dual role as a biomarker and hepatic-derived transporter to target tissues. SELENOP expression is tightly modulated by dietary selenium availability, inflammatory signals, hypoxic conditions, and pharmacological agents. However, comprehensive pharmacological screening to identify regulatory compounds remains unexplored [118]. Current therapeutic strategies for muscle-related disorders lack targeted delivery systems. Advances in nanotechnology, however, have enabled the development of nanoparticle-based drug carriers (e.g., nanoscale delivery platforms) that demonstrate potential for tissue-specific targeting. Notably, calcium-incorporated nanoparticles designed to regulate calcium homeostasis have recently emerged as promising tools for modulating the bone microenvironment and attenuating pathological progression [119]. Similarly, selenium nanomodulation may be used to treat muscle diseases one day.

6.2. Synergistic Effects of Selenium with Other Trace Elements

Vitamin E (α-tocopherol) deficiency commonly coexists with selenium insufficiency. Notably, combined selenium and vitamin E deficiency serves as the predominant etiological factor in most documented myopathic syndromes. Experimental evidence indicates that concurrent selenium and vitamin E deficiency triggers systemic fatal myopathy in guinea pigs, whereas isolated deficiency of either micronutrient leads to attenuated pathological severity [120]. Lipid peroxidation was detected in affected muscle tissues concomitant with reduced GPx activity—a biomarker likely indicative of selenium deficiency. Furthermore, calves fed a selenium-deficient diet supplemented with adequate tocopherol and low polyunsaturated fatty acids [121] exhibited no myopathic manifestations. These findings suggest vitamin E may exacerbate the pathological consequences of selenium deficiency, though the mechanistic interplay remains unresolved [30]. Synergistic micronutrient supplementation strategies combining selenium and vitamin E have been employed to enhance antioxidant enzyme activity and improve endurance performance. Recent clinical trials demonstrated that the co-administration of selenium (17.5 μg/day as sodium selenite) and vitamin E (400 IU/day) significantly lowered post-exercise malondialdehyde (MDA) and lactate dehydrogenase (LDH) levels while elevating superoxide dismutase (SOD) and GPx activities compared to placebo ($p < 0.05$) [101–103].

6.3. Gut-Muscle Axis and Regulation of Selenium

Given that dietary selenium supplements are ingested and absorbed in the intestine, a gut microbiota–muscle axis may mediate selenium's effects on skeletal muscle health. This axis potentially links microbial communities to exercise performance, muscle strength maintenance, and the prevention of motor function decline. Emerging evidence indicates that microbiota–muscle crosstalk and microbiota–mitochondrial communication modulate age-related muscle dysfunction. Specifically, the gut microbiota–muscle axis operates via the modulation of metabolic pathways and mitochondrial network dynamics in skeletal muscle, with dynamin-related protein 1 (DRP1)—a key regulator of mitochondrial fission—being essential to mitigate exercise capacity deterioration during aging [122].

7. Conclusions

Selenium plays a multifunctional role in preserving skeletal muscle homeostasis and enhancing exercise capacity through three primary mechanisms: antioxidative defense mechanisms, the precise regulation of selenoprotein biosynthesis, and the orchestrated modulation of redox-sensitive signaling pathways. Current mechanistic investigations remain predominantly confined to preclinical animal models, highlighting an imperative need for well-designed human clinical trials to validate these preclinical findings and establish causal relationships. The strategic integration of optimized selenium supplementation with evidence-based exercise protocols emerges as a promising intervention for mitigating age-related muscle decline and preventing exercise-induced musculoskeletal injuries. Future research priorities should focus on three translational dimensions: (1) dose–response optimization through pharmacokinetic/pharmacodynamic modeling, (2) systems-level elucidation of selenoprotein–muscle interactome networks, and (3) clinical validation of selenium's ergogenic potential via randomized controlled trials, ultimately enabling targeted applications in sports nutrition and preventive medicine.

Author Contributions: Conceptualization, W.Z. and K.Z.; methodology, K.Z.; validation, W.Z. and K.Z.; data curation, Q.W. and K.Z.; writing—original draft preparation, Q.W. and J.H.; writing—review and editing, Q.W.; visualization, J.H.; supervision, W.Z. and K.Z.; project administration, K.Z.; All authors have read and agreed to the published version of the manuscript.

Funding: This research received no external funding.

Conflicts of Interest: The authors declare no conflict of interest.

References

1. Han, S.-J.; Lee, B.C.; Yim, S.H.; Gladyshev, V.N.; Lee, S.-R. Characterization of Mammalian Selenoprotein O: A Redox-Active Mitochondrial Protein. *PLoS ONE* **2014**, *9*, e95518. [CrossRef]
2. Johansson, L.; Gafvelin, G.; Arnér, E.S.J. Selenocysteine in Proteins—Properties and Biotechnological Use. *Biochim. Biophys. Acta (BBA)-Gen. Subj.* **2005**, *1726*, 1–13. [CrossRef] [PubMed]
3. Rayman, M.P. The Importance of Selenium to Human Health. *Lancet* **2000**, *356*, 233–241. [CrossRef]
4. Köhrle, J. Selenium in Endocrinology-Selenoprotein-Related Diseases, Population Studies, and Epidemiological Evidence. *Endocrinology* **2021**, *162*, bqaa228. [CrossRef]
5. Reeves, M.A.; Hoffmann, P.R. The Human Selenoproteome: Recent Insights into Functions and Regulation. *Cell. Mol. Life Sci.* **2009**, *66*, 2457–2478. [CrossRef] [PubMed]
6. Tsuji, P.A.; Santesmasses, D.; Lee, B.J.; Gladyshev, V.N.; Hatfield, D.L. Historical Roles of Selenium and Selenoproteins in Health and Development: The Good, the Bad and the Ugly. *Int. J. Mol. Sci.* **2022**, *23*, 5. [CrossRef] [PubMed]
7. Bartholomew, A.; Latshaw, D.; Swayne, D.E. Changes in Blood Chemistry, Hematology, and Histology Caused by a Selenium/Vitamin E Deficiency and Recovery in Chicks. *Biol. Trace Elem. Res.* **1998**, *62*, 7–16. [CrossRef]
8. Wu, H.; Xu, T.; Yang, N.; Zhang, J.; Xu, S. Low-Se Diet Increased Mitochondrial ROS to Suppress Myoblasts Proliferation and Promote Apoptosis in Broilers via miR-365-3p/SelT Signaling Axis. *J. Agric. Food Chem.* **2024**, *72*, 284–299. [CrossRef]
9. Wu, H.; Shi, X.; Yang, N.; Xu, S. Low Selenium Diet Inhibited CaMKII Activation via miR-365-3p/SelT Signaling Axis, Resulting in Myoblast Differentiation Disorders and Skeletal Muscle Damage in Broilers. *Biol. Trace Elem. Res.* **2025**. [CrossRef]
10. Wang, S.; Zhao, X.; Liu, Q.; Wang, Y.; Li, S.; Xu, S. Selenoprotein K Protects Skeletal Muscle from Damage and Is Required for Satellite Cells-Mediated Myogenic Differentiation. *Redox Biol.* **2022**, *50*, 102255. [CrossRef]
11. Dumont, N.A.; Bentzinger, C.F.; Sincennes, M.-C.; Rudnicki, M.A. Satellite Cells and Skeletal Muscle Regeneration. *Compr. Physiol.* **2015**, *5*, 1027–1059. [CrossRef] [PubMed]
12. Jing, J.; He, Y.; Liu, Y.; Tang, J.; Wang, L.; Jia, G.; Liu, G.; Chen, X.; Tian, G.; Cai, J.; et al. Selenoproteins Synergistically Protect Porcine Skeletal Muscle from Oxidative Damage via Relieving Mitochondrial Dysfunction and Endoplasmic Reticulum Stress. *J. Anim. Sci. Biotechnol.* **2023**, *14*, 79. [CrossRef]
13. Pedersen, N.D.; Whanger, P.D.; Weswig, P.H.; Muth, O.H. Selenium Binding Proteins in Tissues of Normal and Selenium Responsive Myopathic Lambs. *Bioinorg. Chem.* **1972**, *2*, 33–45. [CrossRef]
14. Jeong, D.-W.; Kim, T.S.; Chung, Y.W.; Lee, B.J.; Kim, I.Y. Selenoprotein W Is a Glutathione-Dependent Antioxidant in Vivo. *FEBS Lett.* **2002**, *517*, 225–228. [CrossRef]
15. Ko, K.Y.; Lee, J.H.; Jang, J.K.; Jin, Y.; Kang, H.; Kim, I.Y. S-Glutathionylation of Mouse Selenoprotein W Prevents Oxidative Stress-Induced Cell Death by Blocking the Formation of an Intramolecular Disulfide Bond. *Free Radic. Biol. Med.* **2019**, *141*, 362–371. [CrossRef]
16. Hawkes, W.C.; Alkan, Z. Delayed Cell Cycle Progression in Selenoprotein W-Depleted Cells Is Regulated by a Mitogen-Activated Protein Kinase Kinase 4-P38/c-Jun NH2-Terminal Kinase-P53 Pathway. *J. Biol. Chem.* **2012**, *287*, 27371–27379 [CrossRef]
17. Noh, O.J.; Park, Y.H.; Chung, Y.W.; Kim, I.Y. Transcriptional Regulation of Selenoprotein W by MyoD during Early Skeletal Muscle Differentiation. *J. Biol. Chem.* **2010**, *285*, 40496–40507. [CrossRef] [PubMed]
18. Jeon, Y.H.; Park, Y.H.; Lee, J.H.; Hong, J.-H.; Kim, I.Y. Selenoprotein W Enhances Skeletal Muscle Differentiation by Inhibiting TAZ Binding to 14-3-3 Protein. *Biochim. Biophys. Acta* **2014**, *1843*, 1356–1364. [CrossRef]
19. Yang, J.-C.; Liu, M.; Huang, R.-H.; Zhao, L.; Niu, Q.-J.; Xu, Z.-J.; Wei, J.-T.; Lei, X.G.; Sun, L.-H. Loss of SELENOW Aggravates Muscle Loss with Regulation of Protein Synthesis and the Ubiquitin-Proteasome System. *Sci. Adv.* **2024**, *10*, eadj4122. [CrossRef]
20. van Dronkelaar, C.; Fultinga, M.; Hummel, M.; Kruizenga, H.; Weijs, P.J.M.; Tieland, M. Minerals and Sarcopenia in Older Adults: An Updated Systematic Review. *J. Am. Med. Dir. Assoc.* **2023**, *24*, 1163–1172. [CrossRef]
21. Pozzer, D.; Varone, E.; Chernorudskiy, A.; Schiarea, S.; Missiroli, S.; Giorgi, C.; Pinton, P.; Canato, M.; Germinario, E.; Nogara, L.; et al. A Maladaptive ER Stress Response Triggers Dysfunction in Highly Active Muscles of Mice with SELENON Loss. *Redox Biol.* **2019**, *20*, 354–366. [CrossRef] [PubMed]

22. Varone, E.; Pozzer, D.; Di Modica, S.; Chernorudskiy, A.; Nogara, L.; Baraldo, M.; Cinquanta, M.; Fumagalli, S.; Villar-Quiles, R.N.; De Simoni, M.-G.; et al. SELENON (SEPN1) Protects Skeletal Muscle from Saturated Fatty Acid-Induced ER Stress and Insulin Resistance. *Redox Biol.* **2019**, *24*, 101176. [CrossRef] [PubMed]
23. Jurynec, M.J.; Xia, R.; Mackrill, J.J.; Gunther, D.; Crawford, T.; Flanigan, K.M.; Abramson, J.J.; Howard, M.T.; Grunwald, D.J. Selenoprotein N Is Required for Ryanodine Receptor Calcium Release Channel Activity in Human and Zebrafish Muscle. *Proc. Natl. Acad. Sci. USA* **2008**, *105*, 12485–12490. [CrossRef] [PubMed]
24. Fomenko, D.E.; Gladyshev, V.N. CxxS: Fold-Independent Redox Motif Revealed by Genome-Wide Searches for Thiol/Disulfide Oxidoreductase Function. *Protein Sci.* **2002**, *11*, 2285–2296. [CrossRef]
25. Deniziak, M.; Thisse, C.; Rederstorff, M.; Hindelang, C.; Thisse, B.; Lescure, A. Loss of Selenoprotein N Function Causes Disruption of Muscle Architecture in the Zebrafish Embryo. *Exp. Cell Res.* **2007**, *313*, 156–167. [CrossRef] [PubMed]
26. Fodor, J.; Al-Gaadi, D.; Czirják, T.; Oláh, T.; Dienes, B.; Csernoch, L.; Szentesi, P. Improved Calcium Homeostasis and Force by Selenium Treatment and Training in Aged Mouse Skeletal Muscle. *Sci. Rep.* **2020**, *10*, 1707. [CrossRef]
27. Lescure, A.; Rederstorff, M.; Krol, A.; Guicheney, P.; Allamand, V. Selenoprotein Function and Muscle Disease. *Biochim. Biophys. Acta (BBA)-Gen. Subj.* **2009**, *1790*, 1569–1574. [CrossRef]
28. Yao, H.; Fan, R.; Zhao, X.; Zhao, W.; Liu, W.; Yang, J.; Sattar, H.; Zhao, J.; Zhang, Z.; Xu, S. Selenoprotein W Redox-Regulated Ca^{2+} Channels Correlate with Selenium Deficiency-Induced Muscles Ca^{2+} Leak. *Oncotarget* **2016**, *7*, 57618–57632. [CrossRef]
29. Chen, X.-W.; Li, Y.; Fu, Y.-T.; Xu, W.-X.; Yang, J.; Wen, X.; Fan, R.-F. Down-Regulation of Selenoprotein K Impairs the Proliferation and Differentiation of Chicken Skeletal Muscle Satellite Cells by Inhibiting the Nrf2 Antioxidant Signaling Pathway. *Free Radic. Res.* **2025**, *59*, 215–225. [CrossRef]
30. Rederstorff, M.; Krol, A.; Lescure, A. Understanding the Importance of Selenium and Selenoproteins in Muscle Function. *Cell. Mol. Life Sci.* **2006**, *63*, 52–59. [CrossRef]
31. Kim, C.Y.; Kim, K.-H. Dexamethasone-Induced Selenoprotein S Degradation Is Required for Adipogenesis. *J. Lipid Res.* **2013**, *54*, 2069–2082. [CrossRef]
32. Fradejas, N.; Serrano-Pérez, M.D.C.; Tranque, P.; Calvo, S. Selenoprotein S Expression in Reactive Astrocytes Following Brain Injury. *Glia* **2011**, *59*, 959–972. [CrossRef] [PubMed]
33. Du, S.; Liu, H.; Huang, K. Influence of SelS Gene Silence on Beta-Mercaptoethanol-Mediated Endoplasmic Reticulum Stress and Cell Apoptosis in HepG2 Cells. *Biochim. Biophys. Acta* **2010**, *1800*, 511–517. [CrossRef] [PubMed]
34. He, L.; Wang, B.; Yao, Y.; Su, M.; Ma, H.; Jia, N. Protective Effects of the SEPS1 Gene on Lipopolysaccharide-Induced Sepsis. *Mol. Med. Rep.* **2014**, *9*, 1869–1876. [CrossRef] [PubMed]
35. Allamand, V.; Richard, P.; Lescure, A.; Ledeuil, C.; Desjardin, D.; Petit, N.; Gartioux, C.; Ferreiro, A.; Krol, A.; Pellegrini, N.; et al. A Single Homozygous Point Mutation in a 3′untranslated Region Motif of Selenoprotein N mRNA Causes SEPN1-Related Myopathy. *EMBO Rep.* **2006**, *7*, 450–454. [CrossRef]
36. Wright, C.R.; Allsopp, G.L.; Addinsall, A.B.; McRae, N.L.; Andrikopoulos, S.; Stupka, N. A Reduction in Selenoprotein S Amplifies the Inflammatory Profile of Fast-Twitch Skeletal Muscle in the Mdx Dystrophic Mouse. *Mediat. Inflamm.* **2017**, *2017*, 7043429. [CrossRef]
37. Powers, S.K.; Lennon, S.L. Analysis of Cellular Responses to Free Radicals: Focus on Exercise and Skeletal Muscle. *Proc. Nutr. Soc.* **1999**, *58*, 1025–1033. [CrossRef]
38. Tessier, F.; Hida, H.; Favier, A.; Marconnet, P. Muscle GSH-Px Activity after Prolonged Exercise, Training, and Selenium Supplementation. *Biol. Trace Elem. Res.* **1995**, *47*, 279–285. [CrossRef]
39. Czyżowska, A.; Brown, J.; Xu, H.; Sataranatarajan, K.; Kinter, M.; Tyrell, V.J.; O'Donnell, V.B.; Van Remmen, H. Elevated Phospholipid Hydroperoxide Glutathione Peroxidase (GPX4) Expression Modulates Oxylipin Formation and Inhibits Age-Related Skeletal Muscle Atrophy and Weakness. *Redox Biol.* **2023**, *64*, 102761. [CrossRef]
40. Schnurr, K.; Belkner, J.; Ursini, F.; Schewe, T.; Kühn, H. The Selenoenzyme Phospholipid Hydroperoxide Glutathione Peroxidase Controls the Activity of the 15-Lipoxygenase with Complex Substrates and Preserves the Specificity of the Oxygenation Products. *J. Biol. Chem.* **1996**, *271*, 4653–4658. [CrossRef]
41. Patterson, A.D.; Carlson, B.A.; Li, F.; Bonzo, J.A.; Yoo, M.-H.; Krausz, K.W.; Conrad, M.; Chen, C.; Gonzalez, F.J.; Hatfield, D.L. Disruption of Thioredoxin Reductase 1 Protects Mice from Acute Acetaminophen-Induced Hepatotoxicity through Enhanced NRF2 Activity. *Chem. Res. Toxicol.* **2013**, *26*, 1088–1096. [CrossRef] [PubMed]
42. Blottner, D.; Moriggi, M.; Trautmann, G.; Furlan, S.; Block, K.; Gutsmann, M.; Torretta, E.; Barbacini, P.; Capitanio, D.; Rittweger, J.; et al. Nitrosative Stress in Astronaut Skeletal Muscle in Spaceflight. *Antioxidants* **2024**, *13*, 432. [CrossRef] [PubMed]
43. Kiermayer, C.; Michalke, B.; Schmidt, J.; Brielmeier, M. Effect of Selenium on Thioredoxin Reductase Activity in Txnrd1 or Txnrd2 Hemizygous Mice. *Biol. Chem.* **2007**, *388*, 1091–1097. [CrossRef]
44. Zhong, Y.; Liu, J.; Cheng, X.; Zhang, H.; Zhang, C.; Xia, Z.; Wu, Z.; Zhang, L.; Zheng, Y.; Gao, Z.; et al. Design, Synthesis and Biological Evaluations of Diverse Michael Acceptor-Based Phenazine Hybrid Molecules as TrxR1 Inhibitors. *Bioorg. Chem.* **2021**, *109*, 104736. [CrossRef]

45. Fu, Y.; Wang, Y.; Bu, Q.; Guo, M. Selenium Deficiency Caused Fibrosis as an Oxidative Stress-Induced Inflammatory Injury in the Lungs of Mice. *Biol. Trace Elem. Res.* **2022**, *201*, 1286–1300. [CrossRef]
46. Kaya, A.; Lee, B.C.; Gladyshev, V.N. Regulation of Protein Function by Reversible Methionine Oxidation and the Role of Selenoprotein MsrB1. *Antioxid. Redox Signal.* **2015**, *23*, 814–822. [CrossRef] [PubMed]
47. Fomenko, D.E.; Novoselov, S.V.; Natarajan, S.K.; Lee, B.C.; Koc, A.; Carlson, B.A.; Lee, T.-H.; Kim, H.-Y.; Hatfield, D.L.; Gladyshev, V.N. MsrB1 (Methionine-R-Sulfoxide Reductase 1) Knock-out Mice. *J. Biol. Chem.* **2009**, *284*, 5986–5993. [CrossRef]
48. Ren, B.; Liu, M.; Ni, J.; Tian, J. Role of Selenoprotein F in Protein Folding and Secretion: Potential Involvement in Human Disease. *Nutrients* **2018**, *10*, 1619. [CrossRef]
49. Jia, S.-Z.; Xu, X.-W.; Zhang, Z.-H.; Chen, C.; Chen, Y.-B.; Huang, S.-L.; Liu, Q.; Hoffmann, P.R.; Song, G.-L. Selenoprotein K Deficiency-Induced Apoptosis: A Role for Calpain and the ERS Pathway. *Redox Biol.* **2021**, *47*, 102154. [CrossRef]
50. Du, S.; Zhou, J.; Jia, Y.; Huang, K. SelK Is a Novel ER Stress-Regulated Protein and Protects HepG2 Cells from ER Stress Agent-Induced Apoptosis. *Arch. Biochem. Biophys.* **2010**, *502*, 137–143. [CrossRef]
51. Gong, T.; Hashimoto, A.C.; Sasuclark, A.R.; Khadka, V.S.; Gurary, A.; Pitts, M.W. Selenoprotein M Promotes Hypothalamic Leptin Signaling and Thioredoxin Antioxidant Activity. *Antioxid. Redox Signal.* **2021**, *35*, 775–787. [CrossRef] [PubMed]
52. Huang, J.; Bao, D.; Lei, C.-T.; Tang, H.; Zhang, C.-Y.; Su, H.; Zhang, C. Selenoprotein T Protects against Cisplatin-Induced Acute Kidney Injury through Suppression of Oxidative Stress and Apoptosis. *FASEB J.* **2020**, *34*, 11983–11996. [CrossRef] [PubMed]
53. Abid, H.; Cartier, D.; Hamieh, A.; François-Bellan, A.-M.; Bucharles, C.; Pothion, H.; Manecka, D.-L.; Leprince, J.; Adriouch, S.; Boyer, O.; et al. AMPK Activation of PGC-1α/NRF-1-Dependent SELENOT Gene Transcription Promotes PACAP-Induced Neuroendocrine Cell Differentiation Through Tolerance to Oxidative Stress. *Mol. Neurobiol.* **2019**, *56*, 4086–4101. [CrossRef] [PubMed]
54. Rocca, C.; De Bartolo, A.; Granieri, M.C.; Rago, V.; Amelio, D.; Falbo, F.; Malivindi, R.; Mazza, R.; Cerra, M.C.; Boukhzar, L.; et al. The Antioxidant Selenoprotein T Mimetic, PSELT, Induces Preconditioning-like Myocardial Protection by Relieving Endoplasmic-Reticulum Stress. *Antioxidants* **2022**, *11*, 571. [CrossRef]
55. Grumolato, L.; Ghzili, H.; Montero-Hadjadje, M.; Gasman, S.; Lesage, J.; Tanguy, Y.; Galas, L.; Ait-Ali, D.; Leprince, J.; Guérineau, N.C.; et al. Selenoprotein T Is a PACAP-Regulated Gene Involved in Intracellular Ca^{2+} Mobilization and Neuroendocrine Secretion. *FASEB J.* **2008**, *22*, 1756–1768. [CrossRef]
56. Guo, Q.; Li, Z.-F.; Hu, D.-Y.; Li, P.-J.; Wu, K.-N.; Fan, H.-H.; Deng, J.; Wu, H.-M.; Zhang, X.; Zhu, J.-H. The Selenocysteine-Containing Protein SELENOT Maintains Dopamine Signaling in the Midbrain to Protect Mice from Hyperactivity Disorder. *EMBO J.* **2025**, *44*, 2906–2927. [CrossRef]
57. Wesolowski, L.T.; Semanchik, P.L.; White-Springer, S.H. Beyond Antioxidants: Selenium and Skeletal Muscle Mitochondria. *Front. Vet. Sci.* **2022**, *9*, 1011159. [CrossRef]
58. Bouman, K.; Groothuis, J.T.; Doorduin, J.; van Alfen, N.; Udink Ten Cate, F.E.A.; van den Heuvel, F.M.A.; Nijveldt, R.; Kamsteeg, E.-J.; Dittrich, A.T.M.; Draaisma, J.M.T.; et al. SELENON-Related Myopathy Across the Life Span, a Cross-Sectional Study for Preparing Trial Readiness. *J. Neuromuscul. Dis.* **2023**, *10*, 1055–1074. [CrossRef]
59. Castets, P.; Lescure, A.; Guicheney, P.; Allamand, V. Selenoprotein N in Skeletal Muscle: From Diseases to Function. *J. Mol. Med.* **2012**, *90*, 1095–1107. [CrossRef]
60. Chernorudskiy, A.; Varone, E.; Colombo, S.F.; Fumagalli, S.; Cagnotto, A.; Cattaneo, A.; Briens, M.; Baltzinger, M.; Kuhn, L.; Bachi, A.; et al. Selenoprotein N Is an Endoplasmic Reticulum Calcium Sensor That Links Luminal Calcium Levels to a Redox Activity. *Proc. Natl. Acad. Sci. USA* **2020**, *117*, 21288–21298. [CrossRef]
61. Misu, H.; Takayama, H.; Saito, Y.; Mita, Y.; Kikuchi, A.; Ishii, K.; Chikamoto, K.; Kanamori, T.; Tajima, N.; Lan, F.; et al. Deficiency of the Hepatokine Selenoprotein P Increases Responsiveness to Exercise in Mice through Upregulation of Reactive Oxygen Species and AMP-Activated Protein Kinase in Muscle. *Nat. Med.* **2017**, *23*, 508–516. [CrossRef] [PubMed]
62. Saito, Y. Selenium Transport Mechanism via Selenoprotein P-Its Physiological Role and Related Diseases. *Front. Nutr.* **2021**, *8*, 685517. [CrossRef]
63. Lee, J.H.; Kwon, J.H.; Jeon, Y.H.; Ko, K.Y.; Lee, S.-R.; Kim, I.Y. Pro178 and Pro183 of Selenoprotein S Are Essential Residues for Interaction with P97(VCP) during Endoplasmic Reticulum-Associated Degradation. *J. Biol. Chem.* **2014**, *289*, 13758–13768. [CrossRef]
64. Sun, S.; Shi, G.; Han, X.; Francisco, A.B.; Ji, Y.; Mendonça, N.; Liu, X.; Locasale, J.W.; Simpson, K.W.; Duhamel, G.E.; et al. Sel1L Is Indispensable for Mammalian Endoplasmic Reticulum-Associated Degradation, Endoplasmic Reticulum Homeostasis, and Survival. *Proc. Natl. Acad. Sci. USA* **2014**, *111*, E582–E591. [CrossRef]
65. Shi, Z.; Han, Z.; Chen, J.; Zhou, J.-C. Endoplasmic Reticulum-Resident Selenoproteins and Their Roles in Glucose and Lipid Metabolic Disorders. *Biochim. Biophys. Acta (BBA)-Mol. Basis Dis.* **2024**, *1870*, 167246. [CrossRef]
66. Wang, S.; Tian, B.; Hu, Y.; Li, T.; Cui, X.; Zhang, L.; Luo, X. Research Progress on the Biological Regulatory Mechanisms of Selenium on Skeletal Muscle in Broilers. *Poult. Sci.* **2024**, *103*, 103646. [CrossRef]

67. Handy, D.E.; Loscalzo, J. The Role of Glutathione Peroxidase-1 in Health and Disease. *Free Radic. Biol. Med.* **2022**, *188*, 146–161. [CrossRef] [PubMed]
68. Xie, Y.; Kang, R.; Klionsky, D.J.; Tang, D. GPX4 in Cell Death, Autophagy, and Disease. *Autophagy* **2023**, *19*, 2621–2638. [CrossRef] [PubMed]
69. Barage, S.H.; Deobagkar, D.D.; Baladhye, V.B. Characterization of Structural and Functional Role of Selenocysteine in Selenoprotein H and Its Impact on DNA Binding. *Amino Acids* **2018**, *50*, 593–607. [CrossRef]
70. Salvatore, D.; Simonides, W.S.; Dentice, M.; Zavacki, A.M.; Larsen, P.R. Thyroid Hormones and Skeletal Muscle--New Insights and Potential Implications. *Nat. Rev. Endocrinol.* **2014**, *10*, 206–214. [CrossRef]
71. Carmody, C.; Ogawa-Wong, A.N.; Martin, C.; Luongo, C.; Zuidwijk, M.; Sager, B.; Petersen, T.; Roginski Guetter, A.; Janssen, R.; Wu, E.Y.; et al. A Global Loss of Dio2 Leads to Unexpected Changes in Function and Fiber Types of Slow Skeletal Muscle in Male Mice. *Endocrinology* **2019**, *160*, 1205–1222. [CrossRef] [PubMed]
72. Lin, S.; Chen, C.; Ouyang, P.; Cai, Z.; Liu, X.; Abdurahman, A.; Peng, J.; Li, Y.; Zhang, Z.; Song, G.-L. SELENOM Knockout Induces Synaptic Deficits and Cognitive Dysfunction by Influencing Brain Glucose Metabolism. *J. Agric. Food Chem.* **2023**, *71*, 1607–1619. [CrossRef] [PubMed]
73. Dayal, A.; Schrötter, K.; Pan, Y.; Föhr, K.; Melzer, W.; Grabner, M. The Ca^{2+} Influx through the Mammalian Skeletal Muscle Dihydropyridine Receptor Is Irrelevant for Muscle Performance. *Nat. Commun.* **2017**, *8*, 475. [CrossRef] [PubMed]
74. Oliver, S.R.; Anderson, K.J.; Hunstiger, M.M.; Andrews, M.T. Turning down the Heat: Down-Regulation of Sarcolipin in a Hibernating Mammal. *Neurosci. Lett.* **2019**, *696*, 13–19. [CrossRef]
75. Kumar, A.; Davuluri, G.; Welch, N.; Kim, A.; Gangadhariah, M.; Allawy, A.; Priyadarshini, A.; McMullen, M.R.; Sandlers, Y.; Willard, B.; et al. Oxidative Stress Mediates Ethanol-Induced Skeletal Muscle Mitochondrial Dysfunction and Dysregulated Protein Synthesis and Autophagy. *Free. Radic. Biol. Med.* **2019**, *145*, 284–299. [CrossRef]
76. Shenoy, P.S.; Sen, U.; Kapoor, S.; Ranade, A.V.; Chowdhury, C.R.; Bose, B. Sodium Fluoride Induced Skeletal Muscle Changes: Degradation of Proteins and Signaling Mechanism. *Environ. Pollut.* **2019**, *244*, 534–548. [CrossRef]
77. Savory, L.A.; Kerr, C.J.; Whiting, P.; Finer, N.; McEneny, J.; Ashton, T. Selenium Supplementation and Exercise: Effect on Oxidant Stress in Overweight Adults. *Obesity* **2012**, *20*, 794–801. [CrossRef]
78. Carafoli, E.; Gamble, R.L.; Lehninger, A.L. K^+-Dependent Rebounds and Oscillations in Respiration-Linked Movements of Ca^{++} and H^+ in Rat Liver Mitochondria. *Biochem. Biophys. Res. Commun.* **1965**, *21*, 488–493. [CrossRef]
79. Sogl, B.; Gellissen, G.; Wiesner, R.J. Biogenesis of Giant Mitochondria during Insect Flight Muscle Development in the Locust, *Locusta migratoria* (L.). *Eur. J. Biochem.* **2000**, *267*, 11–17. [CrossRef]
80. Wang, J.; Chen, M.; You, Y.; Guo, J.; Cai, F.; Pi, F.; Ma, L.; Chen, T. Selenium Electrophilic Center Shuttles Active Electrons to Boost Mitochondrial Electron Leakage. *Cell Biomater.* **2025**, *1*, 100010. [CrossRef]
81. Wang, L.; Yin, J.-J.; Zhang, F.; Yu, H.-D.; Chen, F.-F.; Zhang, Z.-Y.; Zhang, X.-Z. Selenium Status Affects Hypertrophic Growth of Skeletal Muscle in Growing Zebrafish by Mediating Protein Turnover. *J. Nutr.* **2021**, *151*, 1791–1801. [CrossRef] [PubMed]
82. Bilodeau, P.A.; Coyne, E.S.; Wing, S.S. The Ubiquitin Proteasome System in Atrophying Skeletal Muscle: Roles and Regulation. *Am. J. Physiol. Cell Physiol.* **2016**, *311*, C392–C403. [CrossRef] [PubMed]
83. Milan, G.; Romanello, V.; Pescatore, F.; Armani, A.; Paik, J.-H.; Frasson, L.; Seydel, A.; Zhao, J.; Abraham, R.; Goldberg, A.L.; et al. Regulation of Autophagy and the Ubiquitin-Proteasome System by the FoxO Transcriptional Network during Muscle Atrophy. *Nat. Commun.* **2015**, *6*, 6670. [CrossRef]
84. Lu, J.; McKinsey, T.A.; Zhang, C.-L.; Olson, E.N. Regulation of Skeletal Myogenesis by Association of the MEF2 Transcription Factor with Class II Histone Deacetylases. *Mol. Cell* **2000**, *6*, 233–244. [CrossRef]
85. Taylor, M.V.; Hughes, S.M. Mef2 and the Skeletal Muscle Differentiation Program. *Semin. Cell Dev. Biol.* **2017**, *72*, 33–44. [CrossRef] [PubMed]
86. Bennett, A.M.; Tonks, N.K. Regulation of Distinct Stages of Skeletal Muscle Differentiation by Mitogen-Activated Protein Kinases. *Science* **1997**, *278*, 1288–1291. [CrossRef]
87. Zetser, A.; Frank, D.; Bengal, E. MAP Kinase Converts MyoD into an Instructive Muscle Differentiation Factor in Xenopus. *Dev. Biol.* **2001**, *240*, 168–181. [CrossRef]
88. Agell, N.; Bachs, O.; Rocamora, N.; Villalonga, P. Modulation of the Ras/Raf/MEK/ERK Pathway by Ca^{2+}, and Calmodulin. *Cell. Signal.* **2002**, *14*, 649–654. [CrossRef]
89. Zhou, J.; Dhakal, K.; Yi, J. Mitochondrial Ca^{2+} Uptake in Skeletal Muscle Health and Disease. *Sci. China Life Sci.* **2016**, *59*, 770–776. [CrossRef]
90. Rezaee, N.; Rahmani-Nia, F.; Delfan, M.; Ghahremani, R. Exercise Training and Probiotic Supplementation Effects on Skeletal Muscle Apoptosis Prevention in Type-I Diabetic Rats. *Life Sci.* **2021**, *285*, 119973. [CrossRef]
91. Nihashi, Y.; Umezawa, K.; Shinji, S.; Hamaguchi, Y.; Kobayashi, H.; Kono, T.; Ono, T.; Kagami, H.; Takaya, T. Distinct Cell Proliferation, Myogenic Differentiation, and Gene Expression in Skeletal Muscle Myoblasts of Layer and Broiler Chickens. *Sci. Rep.* **2019**, *9*, 16527. [CrossRef]

92. Bao, B.; Kang, Z.; Zhang, Y.; Li, K.; Xu, R.; Guo, M. Selenium Deficiency Leads to Reduced Skeletal Muscle Cell Differentiation by Oxidative Stress in Mice. *Biol. Trace Elem. Res.* **2023**, *201*, 1878–1887. [CrossRef] [PubMed]
93. Chariot, P.; Bignani, O. Skeletal Muscle Disorders Associated with Selenium Deficiency in Humans. *Muscle Nerve* **2003**, *27*, 662–668. [CrossRef] [PubMed]
94. Wangdi, J.T.; O'Leary, M.F.; Kelly, V.G.; Jackman, S.R.; Tang, J.C.Y.; Dutton, J.; Bowtell, J.L. Tart Cherry Supplement Enhances Skeletal Muscle Glutathione Peroxidase Expression and Functional Recovery after Muscle Damage. *Med. Sci. Sports Exerc.* **2022**, *54*, 609–621. [CrossRef]
95. McClean, C.; Davison, G.W. Circadian Clocks, Redox Homeostasis, and Exercise: Time to Connect the Dots? *Antioxidants* **2022**, *11*, 256. [CrossRef]
96. Clemente-Suárez, V.J.; Bustamante-Sanchez, Á.; Mielgo-Ayuso, J.; Martínez-Guardado, I.; Martín-Rodríguez, A.; Tornero-Aguilera, J.F. Antioxidants and Sports Performance. *Nutrients* **2023**, *15*, 2371. [CrossRef] [PubMed]
97. Margaritis, I.; Tessier, F.; Prou, E.; Marconnet, P.; Marini, J.-F. Effects of Endurance Training on Skeletal Muscle Oxidative Capacities with and without Selenium Supplementation. *J. Trace Elem. Med. Biol.* **1997**, *11*, 37–43. [CrossRef]
98. Neek, L.S.; Gaeini, A.A.; Choobineh, S. Effect of Zinc and Selenium Supplementation on Serum Testosterone and Plasma Lactate in Cyclist After an Exhaustive Exercise Bout. *Biol. Trace Elem. Res.* **2011**, *144*, 454–462. [CrossRef]
99. Martínez, P.; Martínez, S.; Mingorance, J.A.; Riera-Sampol, A.; Aguiló, A.; Tauler, P. Gastrointestinal Symptoms and Nutritional Intake among Participants in a Non-Professional Cycling Event. *Eur. J. Appl. Physiol.* **2024**, *125*, 37–48. [CrossRef]
100. Yang, Y.-K. The Effect of Dietary Vitamin E and Selenium on Endurance Exercise Performance and Cell Membrane Damage Index. *Korean J. Sports Med.* **2008**, *17*, 1551–1560.
101. Yang, Y.-K. The Influence of Simultaneous Administration of Selenium and Vitamin E on Antioxidant Enzyme Activity and Lipid Peroxidation. *Phys. Act. Nutr.* **2008**, *12*, 157–162.
102. Yang, Y.-K.; Lee, G.-C.; Wook, C.S. The Effect of Selenium Administration for 3 Weeks on Cardiorespiratory function and Antioxidant Enzyme Activity. *Korean J. Sports Med.* **2008**, *17*, 789–798.
103. Jeong, S.-W.; Choi, C.; ChoiSungKeun; Seok, S.; Yang, Y.-K. The Effect of Vitamin E and Selenium Administration on Antioxidant Enzyme Activity and Blood Fatigue Factor. *Korean J. Sports Med.* **2010**, *19*, 1127–1138.
104. Amirdizaj, V.D.; Mocheshi, S.S. Muscle Injury and Oxidative Stress Following the Use of Selenium Supplements and Exhaustive Aerobic Exercise in Young Physically-Active Females. *J. Kermanshah Univ. Med. Sci.* **2016**, *20*, e69743.
105. Rayman, M.P. Selenium and Human Health. *Lancet* **2012**, *379*, 1256–1268. [CrossRef]
106. Tang, J.; Cao, L.; Jia, G.; Liu, G.; Chen, X.; Tian, G.; Cai, J.; Shang, H.; Zhao, H. The Protective Effect of Selenium from Heat Stress-Induced Porcine Small Intestinal Epithelial Cell Line (IPEC-J2) Injury Is Associated with Regulation Expression of Selenoproteins. *Br. J. Nutr.* **2019**, *122*, 1081–1090. [CrossRef]
107. EFSA Panel on Nutrition, N.F. and F.A. (NDA); Turck, D.; Bohn, T.; Castenmiller, J.; de Henauw, S.; Hirsch-Ernst, K.-I.; Knutsen, H.K.; Maciuk, A.; Mangelsdorf, I.; McArdle, H.J.; et al. Scientific Opinion on the Tolerable Upper Intake Level for Selenium. *EFSA J.* **2023**, *21*, e07704. [CrossRef]
108. Fernández-Lázaro, D.; Fernandez-Lazaro, C.I.; Mielgo-Ayuso, J.; Navascués, L.J.; Córdova Martínez, A.; Seco-Calvo, J. The Role of Selenium Mineral Trace Element in Exercise: Antioxidant Defense System, Muscle Performance, Hormone Response, and Athletic Performance. A Systematic Review. *Nutrients* **2020**, *12*, 1790. [CrossRef]
109. Wen, Y.; Zhang, L.; Li, S.; Wang, T.; Jiang, K.; Zhao, L.; Zhu, Y.; Zhao, W.; Lei, X.; Sharma, M.; et al. Effect of Dietary Selenium Intake on CVD: A Retrospective Cohort Study Based on China Health and Nutrition Survey (CHNS) Data. *Public Health Nutr.* **2024**, *27*, e122. [CrossRef]
110. Effect of Selenium Enriched Eggs on Reducing Oxidative Stress in Sports Women.-All Databases. Available online: https://informaticsjournals.co.in/index.php/ijnd/article/view/4777 (accessed on 23 May 2025).
111. Akil, M.; Gurbuz, U.; Bicer, M.; Sivrikaya, A.; Mogulkoc, R.; Baltaci, A.K. Effect of Selenium Supplementation on Lipid Peroxidation, Antioxidant Enzymes, and Lactate Levels in Rats Immediately After Acute Swimming Exercise. *Biol. Trace Elem. Res.* **2011**, *142*, 651–659. [CrossRef]
112. Selenium Supplementation Prevents Lipid Peroxidation Caused by Arduous Exercise in Rat Brain Tissue—PubMed. Available online: https://pubmed.ncbi.nlm.nih.gov/21692404/ (accessed on 23 May 2025).
113. Romero-Herrera, I.; Nogales, F.; Gallego-López, M.D.C.; Díaz-Castro, J.; Carreras, O.; Ojeda, M.L. Selenium Supplementation via Modulation of Selenoproteins Ameliorates Binge Drinking-Induced Oxidative, Energetic, Metabolic, and Endocrine Imbalance in Adolescent Rats' Skeletal Muscle. *Food Funct.* **2024**, *15*, 7988–8007. [CrossRef] [PubMed]
114. Chen, X.; Zhang, J.; Li, H.; Liu, W.; Xi, Y.; Liu, X. A Comprehensive Comparison of Different Selenium Supplements: Mitigation of Heat Stress and Exercise Fatigue-Induced Liver Injury. *Front. Nutr.* **2022**, *9*, 917349. [CrossRef] [PubMed]
115. Prigol, M.; Luchese, C.; Nogueira, C.W. Antioxidant Effect of Diphenyl Diselenide on Oxidative Stress Caused by Acute Physical Exercise in Skeletal Muscle and Lungs of Mice. *Cell Biochem. Funct.* **2009**, *27*, 216–222. [CrossRef]

16. Kojouri, G.A.; Sharifi, S. Preventing Effects of Nano-Selenium Particles on Serum Concentration of Blood Urea Nitrogen, Creatinine, and Total Protein During Intense Exercise in Donkey. *J. Equine Vet. Sci.* **2013**, *33*, 597–600. [CrossRef]
17. He, G.; Liu, L.; Ahmed, A. Nanoselenium on Aerobic Endurance Exercise Adaptation. *J. Nanomater.* **2022**, *2022*, 2533440. [CrossRef]
18. Hackler, J.; Demircan, K.; Chillon, T.S.; Sun, Q.; Geisler, N.; Schupp, M.; Renko, K.; Schomburg, L. High Throughput Drug Screening Identifies Resveratrol as Suppressor of Hepatic SELENOP Expression. *Redox Biol.* **2023**, *59*, 102592. [CrossRef]
19. Wu, Y.; Sun, B.; Tang, Y.; Shen, A.; Lin, Y.; Zhao, X.; Li, J.; Monteiro, M.J.; Gu, W. Bone Targeted Nano-Drug and Nano-Delivery. *Bone Res.* **2024**, *12*, 51. [CrossRef]
20. Hill, K.E.; Motley, A.K.; Li, X.; May, J.M.; Burk, R.F. Combined Selenium and Vitamin E Deficiency Causes Fatal Myopathy in Guinea Pigs. *J. Nutr.* **2001**, *131*, 1798–1802. [CrossRef]
21. Hidiroglou, M.; Carson, R.B.; Brossard, G.A. Problems Associated with Selenium Deficiency in Beef Calves. *Can. J. Physiol. Pharmacol.* **1968**, *46*, 853–858. [CrossRef]
22. Dennis, N.; Vazquez-Prada, M.; Xue, F.; Freeman, L.M.; Karamalegos, A.; Kudzminkaite, B.; Brown, I.; Ezcurra, M. A Gut-Microbiota-Muscle Axis That Protects against Age-Related Motor Decline by Regulating Mitochondrial Fission in *C. elegans*. *bioRxiv* **2024**. [CrossRef]

nutrients

Review

Effect of Selenium and Selenoproteins on Radiation Resistance

Shidi Zhang [1], Guowei Zhang [1,2], Pengjie Wang [1], Lianshun Wang [3,*], Bing Fang [1,*] and Jiaqiang Huang [1,*]

1 Beijing Advanced Innovation Center for Food Nutrition and Human Health, Department of Nutrition and Health, China Agricultural University, Beijing 100083, China; sy20233313708@cau.edu.cn (S.Z.); wpj1019@cau.edu.cn (P.W.)
2 Limited Liability Company of Hongda Salt Industry, Hoboksar Mongol Autonomous County, Tacheng 834700, China
3 College of Fisheries and Life Science, Dalian Ocean University, Dalian 116023, China
* Correspondence: wanglianshun@dlou.edu.cn (L.W.); bingfang@cau.edu.cn (B.F.); jqhuang@cau.edu.cn (J.H.)

Abstract: With the advancement of radiological medicine and nuclear industry technology, radiation is increasingly used to diagnose human health disorders. However, large-scale nuclear leakage has heightened concerns about the impact on human organs and tissues. Selenium is an essential trace element that functions in the body mainly in the form of selenoproteins. Selenium and selenoproteins can protect against radiation by stimulating antioxidant actions, DNA repair functions, and immune enhancement. While studies on reducing radiation through antioxidants have been conducted for many years, the underlying mechanisms of selenium and selenoproteins as significant antioxidants in radiation damage mitigation remain incompletely understood. Therefore, this paper aims to provide new insights into developing safe and effective radiation protection agents by summarizing the anti-radiation mechanism of selenium and selenoproteins.

Keywords: selenium; radiation resistance; mechanism

1. Introduction

In recent years, radiation has been widely used in a variety of disciplines, including medical imaging diagnosis, radiotherapy, and radiation sterilization, thereby facilitating the advancement of the medical and food industries. While promoting industrial development, radiation also has some negative effects that cannot be ignored, such as nuclear leakage, medical radiation exposure, and radiation from electronic products. Recently, Japan's nuclear sewage discharge events have increased the risk of radiation to human life, leading to more concerns. Selenium and selenoproteins have attracted the interest of researchers due to their potential in radiation resistance. Studying the effects and mechanisms of selenium and selenoproteins on radiation resistance will help researchers find safer anti-radiation methods and develop effective anti-radiation drugs.

Radiation is categorized into ionizing radiation and non-ionizing radiation. This paper focuses on the damage that ionizing radiation causes to human organs and tissues. Ionizing radiation generates electromagnetic waves of various ions, leading to the production of harmful free radicals in the body, which can result in decreased immunity, skin redness, cancer, and other adverse effects that can cause serious harm and even death [1]. The damage mechanisms can be classified into three types: direct action, indirect action, and bystander effect. Direct damage occurs when high-energy ionizing radiation directly affects important macromolecules with biological activity, such as nuclear DNA, proteins or lipid membranes. The key target of direct damage is DNA, which can result in DNA single-strand and double-strand breaks [2]. Indirect damage is the primary form of ionizing radiation's impact. Ray energy acts on water molecules within cells, causing the ionization of water molecules, producing various reactive oxygen species (ROS), resulting in oxidative stress [3,4]. Under oxidative stress conditions, excessive ROS can cause DNA damage and inhibit DNA repair.

Oligosaccharide molecules in the cell membrane are oxidized to unsaturated free radical dimers, which impair the cell membrane function and cause protein dysfunction. Sustained injury response can affect related signal transduction, such as activation of the p53 signaling pathway, thereby stimulating the expression of cyclin-dependent kinase inhibitors p21 and p16, causing cell senescence [5]. Mitochondrial damage causes a large amount of ROS to escape, induces the loss of mitochondrial respiratory chain complex activity, reduces the efficiency of oxidative phosphorylation level, causes cell apoptosis, leads to mitochondrial cascade damage, and results in the doubling of free radical level in the whole cell, which continues to cause more serious damage [6]. The bystander effect refers to transmitting signals to adjacent or non-irradiated distal cells, causing them to be affected by radiation and exhibit various biological dysfunctions, including DNA damage, chromosomal aberrations, and micronuclei formation [7]. Furthermore, DNA damage and continuous oxidative stress can destabilize growth and secretion in bystander cells. Consequently, the effects induced in bystander cells may even spread to secondary observers and their offspring. Regarding radiation damage mechanisms, existing anti-radiation measures mainly focus on oxidation control, DNA repair enhancement, immune system strengthening, etc. While radio-protective agents appear effective at reducing radiation-induced damage, most synthetic agents have toxic side effects that make them impractical for long-term application. Therefore, searching for new radiation protective measures is very necessary.

Selenium is an essential trace element in the human body and is available in inorganic and organic forms. Inorganic selenium compounds include selenite, elemental selenium, and selenium acids; organic selenium includes selenoproteins, selenomethionine (SeMet), selenium yeast, and selenium polysaccharide. Selenium deficiency in the human body may lead to various diseases [8,9], such as Keshan disease and carbon metabolism disorders, or a decrease in resistance to certain viruses [10,11], and increase in radiation-induced micronucleus formation [12]. Selenium plays various biological functions in the form of selenoproteins in the human body, with 25 distinct species of selenium protein genes identified [13]. Selenoproteins are intracellular antioxidants that play an important role in limiting oxidative damage by acting as oxidoreductases for glutathione peroxidases (GPXs), thioredoxin reductases (TRXRDs), and iodothyronine deiodinases (DIOs). Additionally, several selenoproteins, such as selenoprotein P (SELENOP), selenoprotein H (SELENOH), selenoprotein M, selenoprotein T (SELENOT), and selenoprotein W (SELENOW), possess selenocysteine-like structural domains, suggesting potential redox-related functions [14]. Selenium and selenoproteins have various biological functions. Numerous studies have indicated that selenium exhibits promising anti-tumor effects through its capacity of inhibiting tumor cell development, inducing tumor cells to die, and scavenging reactive oxygen species via selenoproteins [15]. Furthermore, selenium and selenoproteins can enhance immune system regulation [16], heavy metal resistance [17], cardiovascular system protection [18], and radiation resistance. Therefore, selenium and selenoproteins hold promise as potential radio-protective agents.

Selenium and selenoproteins play a crucial role in eliminating free radicals and repairing DNA, thereby contributing to immune regulation and protection against radiation damage. Despite this, there is a lack of comprehensive literature on the anti-radiation properties of selenium and selenoproteins, as well as their underlying mechanisms. Therefore, this review aims to elucidate the anti-radiation effects and mechanisms of selenium and selenoproteins. It also outlines potential prospective future research avenues for their application in anti-radiation therapy.

2. Selenoproteins and Their Anti-Radiation Effects

Ionizing radiation has the potential to cause damage to tissues and may induce cell carcinogenesis. Studies have indicated that selenium and selenoproteins may play a significant role in various stages of radiation-induced damage. Certain selenium compounds can act preventatively during the initial stage of radiation exposure, while others are involved in the regulation, repair, and treatment of tissue damage following exposure to radiation [19].

The following section provides descriptions of selenoproteins with anti-radiation activity, as well as their corresponding effects in mitigating radiation (Table 1).

Table 1. Anti-radiation mechanisms of different selenoproteins.

Selenoprotein	Position	Action Mechanism	Reference
GPX1	Erythrocyte	Eliminate reactive oxygen species to reduce radiation damage; Promote DNA repair to prevent radiation injury; Exert anticancer effects to achieve the treat of radiation damage.	[19–26]
GPX4	Cytoplasm, mitochondria and nucleus	Inhibit lipid peroxidation to reduce radiation damage; Regulate apoptotic markers to alleviate radiation-induced cell apoptosis; Decrease the synthesis of 8-oxo-dG to minimize DNA damage.	[27–30]
SELENOP	Plasma	Inhibition of radiation-induced late reactive oxygen species accumulation; Reduction of tumor occurrence as a tumor suppressor in radiation-induced inflammatory carcinogenesis; Regulation of immune cell function as an antioxidant for immune cells.	[31–37]
SELENOS	Endoplasmic reticulum	Alleviate radiation-induced endoplasmic reticulum stress.	[38,39]
SELENOI	The Golgi apparatus	Plays a crucial role in T cell activation, enhancing the immune response of immune cells.	[40,41]

2.1. Glutathione Peroxidases (GPXs)

The main biological effects of selenium in the human body are mediated by selenoproteins. The glutathione peroxidase (GPX) group is an important component of the selenium protein family, serving as a crucial antioxidant and scavenger of ROS in the body. Furthermore, it regulates the REDOX balance in tissues [20]. Currently, eight GPX isoforms have been found within the GPX family, namely GPX1–GPX8. Among them, GPX1–GPX4 and GPX6 have SeCys as a catalytic site. Thus, they are known as SeCys-containing GPXs. Research has indicated that the molecular functions of GPXs include antioxidant activity, peroxidase activity, and glutathione peroxidase activity. Additionally, GPXS are implicated in glutathione metabolism, arachidonic acid metabolism, and other physiological metabolic processes [21]. Both GPX1 and GPX4 are widely expressed in various tissues and may play a pivotal role in the anti-radiation process. The subsequent content will primarily elaborate the potential anti-radiation pathways of GPX1 and GPX4.

2.1.1. Glutathione Peroxidase 1 (GPX1)

GPX1 is a selenoprotein with an active site containing selenocysteine. It is expressed universally in all tissues and shows high expression levels in red blood cells, liver, lungs, and kidneys. Furthermore, it can be found in cytosol and mitochondria [22]. It plays a crucial role in the cellular antioxidant defense mechanism, and can also promote DNA repair, regulate cardiovascular function, and exhibit anti-cancer activity [23]. Because it is involved in so many biological processes, the essential selenoprotein GPX1 is vital for radiation defense.

GPX1 plays a crucial role in removing the excess free radicals generated by radiation, regulating the REDOX balance in the body, and reducing cell damage caused by radiation, thereby enhancing radiation resistance. Research reports indicate that ROS directly contribute to oxidative stress accumulation and trigger additional ROS production through various mechanisms, further disrupting the body's REDOX balance. According to Diane E. Handy and colleagues, the accumulation of ROS may stimulate REDOX-mediated signal transduction events, including activation of transcription factors such as nuclear factor kappa B (NF-κB), which predominantly occurs in GPx1-deficient endothelial cells and leads to inflammation activation [24]. GPX1 can catalyze the reaction between glutathione (GSH) and some superoxides, to regulate the accumulation of these superoxides. This adjustment helps regulate the generation and accumulation of other forms of ROS, ultimately achieving antioxidant effects [25]. GPX1 also promotes the repair of radiation-induced DNA damage. A study conducted by Morais investigated the changes in selenium levels after exposure to ionizing radiation and H2AX phosphorylation. H2AX is a histone that recruits DNA damage repair proteins to injury sites, and its phosphorylation level indicates the extent of DNA damage repair through its phosphorylation level. The study demonstrated that GPX1 contributes to DNA damage repair [26]. Radiation has the potential to induce tumors and cell carcinogenesis. GPX1 can exert an anticancer effect through various mechanisms. Firstly, it can directly impact specific tumor suppressor genes in cancer cells, such as activating the p53 gene and promoting cancer cell apoptosis. Secondly, it can enhance the sensitivity of tumor cells to chemotherapy drugs [27]. Thirdly, it can inhibit tumorigenesis signaling pathways through antioxidant mechanisms and other means. For example, promoting Nrf2 signaling pathway activation is implicated in tumor prevention, which is considered a primary mechanism of action for many chemopreventive agents in inhibiting tumor formation by preventing ROS-mediated DNA damage [28,29].

2.1.2. Glutathione Peroxidase 4 (GPX4)

Several selenium glutathione peroxidases have been identified to contribute to radiation resistance, with GPX1 and GPX4 being particularly important. Radiation exposure can trigger oxidative stress, leading to potentially severe metabolic dysfunctions such as membrane lipid peroxidation and DNA damage [30]. While GPX4 effectively inhibits lipid peroxide, it also promotes DNA repair to alleviate radiation-induced damage and adverse effects, thereby maximizing its role in radiation therapy.

GPX4 has a more significant function in radiation therapy because, in addition to its efficient inhibition of lipid peroxidation, it also helps repair DNA damage in order to reduce radiation-induced damage and side effects [31]. Within the DNA structure, thymine residues possess the highest electron affinity and are, therefore, the most susceptible sites for free radical injury. GPX4 can reduce thymine peroxide caused by ionizing radiation, reducing DNA damage [32]. Overexpression of GPX4 can totally suppress interleukin-1-induced NF-κB activation, while GPX1 exerted only moderate effects on this pathway [32]. Furthermore, the experimental results demonstrate that GPX4 effectively regulates many apoptosis markers in various cells, such as the release of cytochrome c, DNA fragmentation, and inhibition of NF-κB. For example, it protects the preferred substrate of cytochrome c, cardiolipin, from peroxidation and inhibits the release of cytochrome c from mitochondria in response to oxidative stress exposure, effectively regulating apoptosis [33,34].

2.2. *Selenoprotein P (SELENOP)*

SELENOP is an extracellular glycoprotein, a selenium transporter, and a major supplier of selenium in tissues [35]. It is widely distributed in almost all tissues and it contains ten SeMets, of which the *N*-terminal SeMet have antioxidant functions, while the *C*-terminal nine SeMets are the main suppliers of selenium to tissues. SELENOP also plays a crucial role in certain aspects of immune function. The REDOX tone also influences macrophage differentiation, and several studies have indicated that SELENOP is especially important in this process [36]. Studies suggest that SELENOP is a previously unidentified antioxidant protein capable of regulating the late accumulation of ROS and mitigating toxicity in normal human fibroblasts following radiation exposure. The expression of SELENOP effectively suppresses radiation-induced late ROS accumulation and associated toxicity [37,38]. This indicates that SELENOP is a crucial regulator of the cellular response to radiation. Furthermore, the antioxidant function of SELENOP suggests a possible involvement in cancer prevention, particularly in cases characterized by heightened oxidative stress, such as inflammatory bowel cancer. Research conducted by Caitlyn W. Barrett et al. has demonstrated that SELENOP acts as a haploid tumor suppressor in inflammatory carcinogenesis [39]. At the same time, SELENOP also influences macrophage polarization, reducing the incidence of inflammatory tumors by attenuating the activation of pro-inflammatory cells [39–41].

2.3. Selenoprotein S (SELENOS)

Selenoprotein S (SELENOS) is a small, inherently disordered membrane protein associated with various cellular functions, including inflammatory processes and cellular stress responses. It is most notably recognized for its involvement in the endoplasmic reticulum-associated degradation (ERAD) pathway [42]. This pathway involves the extraction of misfolded proteins or misassembled protein complexes from the endoplasmic reticulum (ER) into the cytosol for proteasomal degradation. Radiation can lead to the accumulation of misfolded proteins in the ER, causing ER stress and triggering the unfolded protein response (UPR), further promoting inflammation. The participation of ERAD SELENOS is crucial in the UPR process, as it regulates the removal of misfolded proteins or incorrectly assembled protein complexes from the ER to the cytoplasm, resulting in proteasomal degradation and alleviating radiation-induced endoplasmic reticulum stress. It is evident that SELENOS is also important in responding to radiation [43].

2.4. Selenoprotein I (SELENOI)

The selenoprotein I (SELENOI) group is a unique among selenoproteins. It acts as an ethanolamine phosphate transferase (Ept) rather than a REDOX catalyst. This enzyme is critical for synthesizing phosphatidyl ethanolamine (PE) and alkenyl PE in pluripotent stem cells, as well as the proliferation of tumor cells [44]. Its involvement in metabolic reprogramming is particularly significant [45]. Selenoprotein I may play crucial functions in T cell activation and metabolic reprogramming. As a component, SELENOI can maintain ethanolamine phospholipid synthesis in cell metabolic reprogramming, thus contributing to the balance of cell metabolism and playing an essential function in the process of T cell activation. Therefore, SELENOI can be instrumental in regulating immune cells to combat radiation-induced immune responses and exhibits radiation resistance [46].

In conclusion, multiple selenoproteins can exert anti-radiation effects through different mechanisms (Figure 1). Glutathione peroxidase 1 (GPX1) and glutathione peroxidase 4 (GPX4) contribute to anti-radiation activities by enhancing DNA repair and regulating anti-inflammatory and anticancer signaling pathways. GPX4 is especially effective at removing lipid peroxidation in response to radiation-induced oxidative stress. GPX1 and SELENOP function by scavenging excess free radicals. GPX4 and SELENOI can also promote radiation-induced apoptosis through immune regulation and other pathways. Meanwhile, SELENOS primarily exerts its anti-radiation activity by relieving endoplasmic reticulum stress.

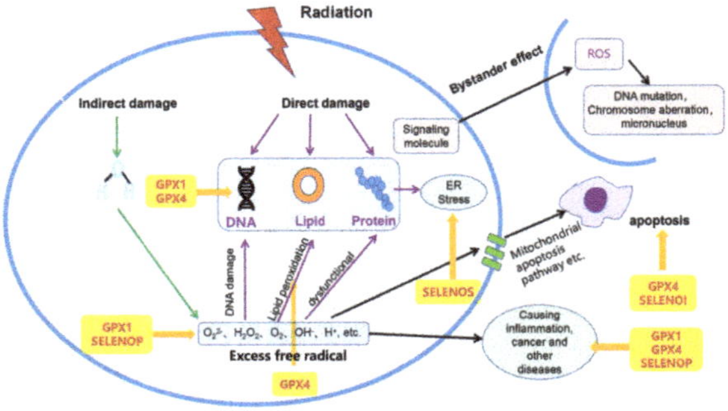

Figure 1. Radiation resistance mechanism of different selenoproteins.

3. Radiation Resistance Mechanism of Selenium and Selenoproteins

Selenium and selenoproteins exhibit the potential to mitigate the effects of radiation, a capability closely linked to biological activities such as anti-oxidation, immune regulation, and apoptosis control. Research has demonstrated that selenium and selenoproteins combat radiation by reducing oxidative damage, regulating the immune system, managing cell apoptosis, and protecting DNA and the hematological system.

3.1. Improves Oxidative Damage

The REDOX system dynamically regulates the production of active oxygen free radicals under normal physiological conditions to maintain a balanced level. Oxidative stress occurs when there is an imbalance between oxidation and anti-oxidation in the body, leading to a pathological condition characterized by high ROS levels [47]. Radiation stimulation causes the ionization and excitation of water molecules, resulting in the generation of an excessive amount of reactive oxygen species. These ROS will subsequently cause a free radical chain reaction, causing oxidative stress. Consequently, excess ROS destroy biological macromolecules such as DNA, lipids, proteins, and mitochondria [3]. Damage to nucleic acids, lipid peroxidation, and protein damage might cause alterations in essential antioxidant enzymes such as SOD and GSH-Px [48]. Additionally, non-enzymatic antioxidants play a crucial role in combating free radicals. These substances include small molecular compounds with antioxidant effects, such as GSH synthesized in cells, ceruloplasmin, and vitamin E [49].

It has been reported that selenium and selenoproteins can scavenge ROS directly. In biological systems, selenium compounds tend to be restored; it is a good nucleophilic reagent. They are used in heavy metal detoxification to produce ROS-required metal ion complexation, which indirectly removes ROS. Selenium also acts as a cofactor for various antioxidant enzymes, such as GSH-Px, and contributes to antioxidant effects [50]. Sodium selenite is the first selenium compound to be studied for radiation protection in a mouse model [51]: it has been shown to be efficient when combined with vitamin E prior to gamma irradiation in mice, preventing the radiation-induced decrease of antioxidant enzymes [52]. Supplementation with sodium selenite has been shown to increase serum GPX activity while decreasing treatment-induced oxidative stress. 3′-3′ Diselendipropionic acid (DSePA) has been identified as a potent radio-protectant. It has shown efficacy as a free radical scavenger, GPX mimic, and anti-hemolytic agent. The high levels of ROS observed in GPX1 knockout mice during the injury response highlight the importance of antioxidant pathways in limiting ROS-induced cell damage [53]. Furthermore, numerous studies have demonstrated that GPX4 regulates lipid peroxidation and cell death induced by radiation. In summary, radiation can induce oxidative stress and pathological changes in the body. Improving oxidative damage is an important mechanism of selenium and selenoproteins against radiation damage.

3.2. Protecting DNA

Thus far, the findings indicate that safeguarding DNA is crucial for selenium and selenium proteins to resist radiation [3]. Ionizing radiation can degrade DNA molecules and damage nucleotides and their components. To overcome this damage, eukaryotes have a DNA repair system in place, which includes processes such as homologous recombination (HR), non-homologous end joining (NHEJ), base excision repair (BER), nucleotide excision repair (NER), and other mechanisms that contribute to DNA repair, genome stability, and aging. Double-stranded DNA breaks are repaired through HR or NHEJ, while single-strand breaks are repaired through BER or NER [54]. Chromosome DNA and protein complexes are sensitive to ionizing radiation, which can stimulate the ionization of cells in inland waters, resulting in a large quantity of reactive oxygen species. The strong oxidizing power of these species can destroy cell DNA, causing double-strand and single-strand breaks that result in chromosome aberrations. A series of in vitro studies, animal models, and human studies have demonstrated that selenium and selenium proteins can prevent DNA damage and enhance the activity of repair enzymes (such as DNA glycosylase, p53, BRCA1, Gadd45) providing protection [55]. GPX1 was shown to stimulate the expression of Gadd45, which is involved in DNA replication and damage repair [56]. SeMet protects against DNA damage by the creation of protein complexes with Ref1, p53, and Brca1. SeMet first induces the DNA repair branch of the p53 pathway. Then, Brca1 and Ref1 simultaneously interact with p53 to form protein complexes that target the induction of DNA repair responses [57].

3.3. Regulating Cell Apoptosis

As a strong stimulus, ionizing radiation can induce cell apoptosis through various mechanisms, including DNA damage, endoplasmic reticulum stress (ER stress), and ROS overload. However, selenium and selenoproteins can exert radio-protective effects by inhibiting cell apoptosis. Research has shown that different forms of selenium have different effects on cell apoptosis, with appropriate doses of selenium nanoparticles being more effective than sodium selenite and yeast selenium [58]. In addition, radiation-induced mitochondrial membrane damage can trigger the ER signaling pathway, ultimately leading to cell apoptosis [59]. Selenoprotein S is a transmembrane protein located in the endoplasmic reticulum (ER) and plasma membrane. It essential in the ER-associated degradation (ERAD) pathway and can regulate ER stress-induced cell apoptosis [60]. Furthermore, studies have indicated that GPX4 inhibits cell apoptosis in vivo through an endogenous apoptotic pathway [33]. This regulatory function is achieved by protecting the preferred substrate, cardiolipin, from oxidation and inhibiting cytochrome c release from mitochondria when exposed to oxidative stress [61,62].

3.4. Regulating Immune System

The immune system, which is made up of immune organs (such as the spleen, thymus, bone marrow, and lymph nodes), immune cells (including lymphocytes, macrophages, and granulocytes), and immune molecules (such as TNF, IFN, and IL), is responsible for preventing pathogens from invading the body and maintaining a healthy body [63]. Studies have shown that selenoproteins, such as selenoprotein I, play a significant role in the activation of T cells [45], while selenoprotein S regulates the steady-state aspects of immunity. This suggests that selenoproteins profoundly affect the activation and regulation of immune cells [64].

3.4.1. MAPK Signaling Pathways and PI3K/AKT Signaling Pathway

Mitogen-activated protein kinase (MAPK) family, which includes extracellular signal-regulated kinase (ERK), p38 mitogen-activated protein kinase, and c-Jun *N*-terminal kinase (JNK). These three essential members participate in cell growth, proliferation, apoptosis, differentiation, and other growth processes [65]. Ionizing radiation stimulates the JNK and P38 pathways, activating classical MAPK signaling pathways and participating in immune regulation [66]. Some studies have shown that selenium deficiency downregulates the expression of 19 selenoproteins, increasing intracellular ROS levels. This, in turn, results in elevated levels of P38 and JNK gene expression, and increased expression of proteins involved in the mitochondrial apoptotic pathway. These findings indicate a close association between selenoproteins and ROS/MAPK-induced apoptosis, particularly necrotic apoptosis. Selenium and selenoproteins can regulate this pathway through multiple targets [67].

The PI3K/AKT pathway is a multifunctional signaling pathway related to defense, cell proliferation, and apoptosis. It regulates mammalian cell development, proliferation, and metabolic regulation. Activation of the PI3K/AKT pathway can accelerate DNA damage repair and inhibit ionizing radiation [68]. Experiments have revealed that hydrogel loaded with selenium nanoparticles (SeNPs) may eliminate reactive oxygen species and modify pH, which may protect cells from oxidative stress. Furthermore, these SeNPs induced macrophage M2 polarization through the PI3K/AKT and MAPK pathways, leading to reduced inflammatory cytokine production—a promising approach for mitigating radiation damage [69].

3.4.2. Inflammation Signaling Pathway

As previously mentioned, exposure to ionizing radiation can lead to extensive oxidative damage, DNA breakage, and cell death. This results in the release of pro-inflammatory cytokines, including IL-1, IL-2, IL-4, IL-6, and TNF-α. Chronic upregulation of these cytokines can result in sustained generation of free radicals and mediate the occurrence of inflammation [70]. Inflammatory cytokines recruit immune cells and regulate the cellular microenvironment. Selenium and selenoproteins also regulate inflammatory factors and signaling pathways as part of their radio-protective mechanisms.

4. The Application of Selenium and Selenoproteins in the Treatment of Radiation-Related Diseases

Exposure to ionizing radiation can result in tissue damage in living organisms. The extent of the damage depends on the radiation exposure level. Acute clinical manifestations can impact the gastrointestinal tract, liver, kidneys, and lungs. Furthermore, organ and tissue damage may also occur. In addition to these organ systems, long-term observations have shown that radiation can also lead to damage to the kidneys, liver, and cardiovascular system, and even result in death [71]. As previously noted, selenium and selenium protein show significant potential in mitigating radiation damage. The selenium compounds used for radioprotection primarily consist of inorganic selenium compounds, selenoamino acids, and selenoproteins. This article will review some of the uses of selenium and selenium protein as radiation protective agents to alleviate multiple organ damage caused by radiation or treat related diseases.

4.1. Lung Injury and Treatment

The lungs are one of the most sensitive organs to ionizing radiation. Aside from cancer radiotherapy, the human body may be exposed to radiation environments for extended periods of time as a result of nuclear or radiation disasters. Lung injury is one of the most dangerous consequences of radiation exposure, which may lead to pneumonia and fibrosis. Severe cases may cause lung cancer and even threaten life [72]. Seleno-L-methionine is an effective antioxidant; previous research demonstrates its enormous potential in protecting and alleviating radiation damage [73]. We can apply seleno-L-methionine to prevent radiation-induced lung toxicity. It can reduce the accumulation of ROS and alleviate radiation-induced DNA damage and cell death by upregulating antioxidant enzymes to eliminate excessive ROS and directly chelating ROS. Amini et al. found that treating rats with seleno-L-methionine reduced the expression of these cytokines, hence reducing macrophage and lymphocyte infiltration [73]. 3′-3′ dithiopropionic acid (DSePA) is a simple, stable, and water-soluble organic selenium compound that can eliminate ROS and exhibits GPX-like activity. DSePA has been found to reduce oxidative damage to tissues by increasing the tissue levels of antioxidant defense enzymes, including GPX, thereby preventing mortality in a whole-body exposed mouse model. Kunwar et al.'s study demonstrated that DSePA treatment can decrease excessive free radicals and lipid peroxidation. This intervention also reduced the severity of pneumonia in mice. It affected the recruitment of lung radiation-induced inflammatory cells, such as pulmonary macrophages and neutrophils, suggesting that DSePA influences the inflammatory cell recruitment involved in the formation of radiation-induced lung injury [74]. SeNPs can prolong the radiation protection time without obvious side effects in the lung. Moreover, they exhibit potent cytotoxicity in cancer cells, but relatively little cytotoxicity in normal healthy cells [75].

4.2. Hematopoietic System

Bone marrow is one of the tissues most sensitive to radiation, and bone damage is a significant cause of death after high-dose irradiation. Studies have shown that prolonged radiation exposure may result in hematopoietic dysfunction, with increased levels of ROS and sustained oxidative stress potentially leading to long-term damage to radiation-induced hematopoietic stem cells (HSC). In an in vivo experiment with sodium selenite in mice, Jian Zhang et al. found that selenium can reduce radiation-induced hematological dysfunction and protect hematopoietic function [76].

4.3. Gastrointestinal System

Long-term radiation exposure can cause tissue damage in the gastrointestinal tract, with persistent oxidative stress potentially leading to inflammatory bowel disease and associated malignancies, most notably colitis [77]. One selenoprotein previously associated with colitis is SELENOP. SELENOP acts as an extracellular antioxidant and serves as a selenium transport protein primarily expressed in the liver and secreted into the plasma. Sarah et al. found that SELENOP deficiency increases the risk of inflammatory cancers, emphasizing the critical antioxidant role of epithelial-produced SELENOP in the colonic milieu [78].

4.4. Kidney and Liver

Following radiation exposure, the kidney tissue generates a large amount of free radicals, leading to oxidative stress, which can result in renal dysfunction or the onset of kidney disease. Both selenite and SeNPs can protect the kidneys from radiation damage by alleviating oxidative injury. However, the data from Karami et al. showed that SeNPs, an emerging agent for delivering selenium, are more effective than selenite [79]. SeNPs also reduced inflammation and edema in irradiated rats, revealing potential anti-inflammatory activity by inhibiting pro-inflammatory genes and antioxidant effects [80].

Ionizing radiation can also induce hepatotoxicity. Studies have shown that SeNPs may have promising applications in mitigating radiation-induced liver toxicity. NF-κB regulates immunological and inflammatory responses, as well as cell apoptosis. Pharmacological inhibition of NF-κB may be a potential approach for treating radiation injuries. SeNPs may reduce hepatotoxicity by stimulating antioxidant status, increasing Nrf2 expression, enhancing GPXs, and reducing pro-inflammatory marker IL6, lowering NF-κB expression [81]. The discussion by Azmoonfar et al. also demonstrates that SeNPs prevent damage to liver tissues induced by infrared and chemical exposure, confirming their liver-protective action [82].

4.5. Cardiovascular System

Cardiovascular diseases account for the majority of global deaths, and radiation-induced cardiovascular disease is one of the main side effects of ionizing radiation exposure. Due to the enormous harm and high mortality caused by cardiovascular damage, it is essential to seek natural and safe therapeutic agents. Amini et al. investigated the combination of selenium-L-methionine and curcumin to determine their capacity to prevent radiation-induced cardiovascular damage. In this study, the combination of selenium-L-methionine and curcumin significantly reduced the expression of pro-inflammatory factors in the heart and blood vessels, indicating its ability to protect cardiovascular health by regulating the redox system and chronic oxidative stress [83]. GPX1 can also repair cardiovascular functional disorders in certain areas. Ye Xiong et al. have found that oxidative stress increases DNA damage, ultimately causing cardiac myocyte cell cycle exit [84]. GPX1 is essential for repairing of cardiovascular damage through DNA repair. Evidence from many other studies indicates that a lack of GPX1 exacerbates heart failure and enhances angiotensin II-mediated cardiac hypertrophy. In contrast, transgenic mice overexpressing GPX1 show higher mitochondrial respiratory efficiency, better contractile strength, and diastolic function compared to wild-type hearts [24,85]. It is evident that GPX1 effectively alleviates cardiovascular damage caused by radiation, protects cardiovascular function, reduces radiation-induced cardiovascular stress, and plays a therapeutic role in radiation treatment.

5. Effects of Selenium and Selenoproteins Doses on Radiation Resistance

The evidence for selenium being a chemoprevention agent includes that from animal and epidemiological studies [86–88]. However, different results regarding the role of selenium and selenoproteins in chemoprevention have emerged, which may be explained by the selenium status entering the experimental subjects as well as the difference in selenium dose [86]. The reviewed studies and some other ongoing investigations have been providing mounting evidence on the beneficial role of selenium in both healthy people and patients, but it is necessary to pay attention to its status, dose, and type. The dose of selenium and selenoproteins associated with anti-radiation effects may be U-shaped; namely, when the selenium content in the human body is less than ideal situation, selenium and selenium protein may play a beneficial role [89], but when the level of selenium in the human body more than is ideal, excessive amounts of selenium and selenium protein may produce adverse effects [90]. For example, a study conducted by Wang et al. on hens supplemented with three different concentrations of selenium orally for three time periods found that excessive intake of selenium led to decreased immunity and increased oxidative damage [91]. In another study, selenium deficiency caused testicular damage and sperm abnormalities during spermatogenesis [92], and selenium excess impaired sperm quality in male rats [93]. This suggested that non-optimal selenium intake decreased sperm quality and quantity by causing the spermatogenic cells loss and shedding in the testes [94]. Selenium concentration changes will destroy the REDOX state and cause oxidative stress, producing adverse effects.

Although the current experimental results of selenium and selenoproteins as chemopreventive agents are inconsistent, most of these experimental studies support the view that there may be a U-shaped correlation between the doses of selenium and selenoproteins and the anti-radiation effect; that is, the optimal intake of selenium can inhibit oxidative stress, inflammation, apoptosis, etc., and achieve anti-oxidation, DNA repair and immunity enhancement. Therefore, it can be concluded that an optimal Se intake will benefit radiation resistance.

6. Summary and Prospects

Selenium is a crucial trace element in the human body, which has great potential for radiation resistance due to its potent antioxidant, DNA repair, and immune regulatory functions. According to current research reports, selenium and selenoproteins enhance antioxidant capacity by clearing hydrogen peroxide and lipid peroxides to combat tissue damage caused by radiation, and exhibit anti-radiation activity through enhancing DNA repair. They protect cells from radiation damage by regulating mitochondrial apoptosis and apoptosis pathways, and also regulate the immune response of the immune system through the MAPK signaling pathway, PI3K/AKT signaling pathway, and inflammatory signaling pathway. Selenium and selenoproteins play an essential role in alleviating and treating radiation damage to organ tissues such as the lungs, kidneys, intestines, cardiovascular systems, etc., with enormous potential.

In the future, we can focus on finding new selenium and selenoproteins with radioprotective functions, and exploring the mechanisms by which different kinds of selenium and selenoproteins work together to protect against radiation. We can also enrich the use of selenium and selenoproteins in multi-organ injury caused by radiation in clinical studies. How to choose the form and dosage of drugs containing selenium will be the challenge. Thus, the complex mechanisms, forms, and dosages of selenium and selenoproteins in anti-radiation activities may become a new research hotspot.

Author Contributions: Conceptualization, S.Z. and J.H.; investigation, S.Z. and G.Z.; visualization, S.Z. and P.W.; writing—original draft preparation, S.Z.; writing—review and editing, S.Z., L.W., B.F. and J.H.; supervision, L.W. and B.F.; funding acquisition, J.H. All authors have read and agreed to the published version of the manuscript.

Funding: This study was supported by the National Natural Science Foundation of China (32172772), the National Key R&D Program of China (No. 2022YFD2101003) and the 111 project from the Education Ministry of China (No. B18053).

Conflicts of Interest: Author Guowei Zhang was employed by the company Limited Liability Company of Hongda Salt Industry. The remaining authors declare that the research was conducted in the absence of any commercial or financial relationships that could be construed as a potential conflict of interest.

Abbreviations

ROS, reactive oxygen species; GPXs, glutathione peroxidases; TXNRDs, thioredoxin reductases; DIOs, iodothyronine deiodinases; SELENOP, selenoprotein P; SELENOH, selenoprotein H; SELENOM, selenoprotein M; SELENOT, selenoprotein T; SELENOW, selenoprotein W; SELENOS, selenoprotein S; SELENOI, selenoprotein I; REDOX, oxidation-reduction; ERAD, endoplasmic reticulum-associated degradation; ER, endoplasmic reticulum; Ept, ethanolamine phosphate transferase; PE, phosphatidyl ethanolamine; SOD, superoxidase dismutase; DSePA, 3′-3′ diselendipropionic acid; HR, recombination; NHEJ, non-homologous end joining; BER, base excision repair; NER, nucleotide excision repair; SeMet, selenomethionine; MAPK, mitogen-activated protein kinase; ERK, extracellular signal-regulated kinase; JNK, c-Jun *N*-terminal kinase; SeNPs, selenium nanoparticles; HSC, hematopoietic stem cells.

References

1. Soule, B.P.; Hyodo, F.; Matsumoto, K.; Simone, N.L.; Cook, J.A.; Krishna, M.C.; Mitchell, J.B. Therapeutic and clinical applications of nitroxide compounds. *Antioxidants Redox Signal.* **2007**, *9*, 1731–1744. [CrossRef]
2. Havránková, R. Biological effects of ionizing radiation. *Cas. Lek. Cesk.* **2020**, *159*, 258–260.
3. Meador, J.A.; Morris, R.J.; Balajee, A.S. Ionizing Radiation-Induced DNA Damage Response in Primary Melanocytes and Keratinocytes of Human Skin. *Cytogenet. Genome Res.* **2022**, *162*, 188–200. [CrossRef] [PubMed]
4. Carante, M.P.; Ramos, R.L.; Ballarini, F. Radiation Damage in Biomolecules and Cells 2.0. *Int. J. Mol. Sci.* **2023**, *24*, 3238. [CrossRef]
5. Ahmed, K.M.; Li, J.J. NF-kappa B-mediated adaptive resistance to ionizing radiation. *Free Radic. Biol Med.* **2008**, *44*, 1–13. [CrossRef]
6. Liu, L.; Liang, Z.; Ma, S.; Li, L.; Liu, X. Radioprotective countermeasures for radiation injury (Review). *Mol. Med. Rep.* **2023**, *27*, 1–14. [CrossRef] [PubMed]
7. Wang, W.; Xue, C.; Mao, X. Radioprotective effects and mechanisms of animal, plant and microbial polysaccharides. *Int. J. Biol. Macromol.* **2020**, *153*, 373–384. [CrossRef] [PubMed]
8. Zhao, L.; Liu, M.; Sun, H.; Yang, J.C.; Huang, Y.X.; Huang, J.Q.; Lei, X.; Sun, L.H. Selenium deficiency-induced multiple tissue damage with dysregulation of immune and redox homeostasis in broiler chicks under heat stress. *Sci. China Life Sci.* **2023**, *66*, 2056–2069. [CrossRef]
9. Li, T.; Zhang, J.; Wang, P.J.; Zhang, Z.W.; Huang, J.Q. Selenoproteins Protect Against Avian Liver Necrosis by Metabolizing Peroxides and Regulating Receptor Interacting Serine Threonine Kinase 1/Receptor Interacting Serine Threonine Kinase 3/Mixed Lineage Kinase Domain-Like and Mitogen-Activated Protein Kinase Signaling. *Front. Physiol.* **2021**, *12*, 696256. [CrossRef]
10. Chen, Y.C.; Prabhu, K.S.; Das, A.; Mastro, A.M. Dietary selenium supplementation modifies breast tumor growth and metastasis. *Int. J. Cancer* **2013**, *133*, 2054–2064. [CrossRef]
11. Yang, J.C.; Huang, Y.X.; Sun, H.; Liu, M.; Zhao, L.; Sun, L.H. Selenium Deficiency Dysregulates One-Carbon Metabolism in Nutritional Muscular Dystrophy of Chicks. *J. Nutr.* **2023**, *153*, 47–55. [CrossRef] [PubMed]
12. Baliga, M.S.; Diwadkar-Navsariwala, V.; Koh, T.; Fayad, R.; Fantuzzi, G.; Diamond, A.M. Selenoprotein deficiency enhances radiation-induced micronuclei formation. *Mol. Nutr. Food Res.* **2008**, *52*, 1300–1304. [CrossRef]
13. Stoytcheva, Z.R.; Berry, M.J. Transcriptional regulation of mammalian selenoprotein expression. *Biochim. Biophys. Acta* **2009**, *1790*, 1429–1440. [CrossRef] [PubMed]
14. Huang, J.; Xie, L.; Song, A.; Zhang, C. Selenium Status and Its Antioxidant Role in Metabolic Diseases. *Oxidative Med. Cell. Longev.* **2022**, *2022*, 7009863. [CrossRef] [PubMed]
15. Kursvietiene, L.; Mongirdiene, A.; Bernatoniene, J.; Sulinskiene, J.; Staneviciene, I. Selenium Anticancer Properties and Impact on Cellular Redox Status. *Antioxidants* **2020**, *9*, 80. [CrossRef]
16. Zhu, K.; Yang, S.; Li, T.; Huang, X.; Dong, Y.; Wang, P.; Huang, J. Advances in the Study of the Mechanism by Which Selenium and Selenoproteins Boost Immunity to Prevent Food Allergies. *Nutrients* **2022**, *14*, 3133. [CrossRef]
17. Sun, H.; Chen, J.; Xiong, D.; Long, M. Detoxification of Selenium Yeast on Mycotoxins and Heavy Metals: A Review. *Biol. Trace Elem. Res.* **2023**, *201*, 5441–5454. [CrossRef]

18. Carroll, L.; Davies, M.J.; Pattison, D.I. Reaction of low-molecular-mass organoselenium compounds (and their sulphur analogues) with inflammation-associated oxidants. *Free Radic. Res.* **2015**, *49*, 750–767. [CrossRef]
19. Farhood, B.; Mortezaee, K.; Motevaseli, E.; Mirtavoos-Mahyari, H.; Shabeeb, D.; Eleojo Musa, A.; Sanikhani, N.S.; Najafi, M.; Ahmadi, A. Selenium as an adjuvant for modification of radiation response. *J. Cell Biochem.* **2019**, *120*, 18559–18571. [CrossRef]
20. Pei, J.; Pan, X.; Wei, G.; Hua, Y. Research progress of glutathione peroxidase family (GPX) in redoxidation. *Front. Pharmacol.* **2023**, *14*, 1147414. [CrossRef]
21. Zhao, Q.; Tang, Y.; Zhang, L.; Sun, N.; Liu, Q.; Zhang, R. Biological Functions of Selenoprotein Glutathione Peroxidases (GPXs) and their Expression in Osteoarthritis. *J. Inflammation Res.* **2023**, *16*, 183–196. [CrossRef] [PubMed]
22. Shimura, T.; Nakashiro, C.; Fujiwara, K.; Shiga, R.; Sasatani, M.; Kamiya, K.; Ushiyama, A. Radiation affects glutathione redox reaction by reduced glutathione peroxidase activity in human fibroblasts. *J. Radia. Res.* **2022**, *63*, 183–191. [CrossRef] [PubMed]
23. Zhao, Y.; Wang, H.; Zhou, J.; Shao, Q. Glutathione Peroxidase GPX1 and Its Dichotomous Roles in Cancer. *Cancers* **2022**, *14*, 2560. [CrossRef]
24. Handy, D.E.; Loscalzo, J. The role of glutathione peroxidase-1 in health and disease. *Free Radic. Biol. Med.* **2022**, *188*, 146–161. [CrossRef]
25. Brigelius-Flohé, R.; Maiorino, M. Glutathione peroxidases. *Biochim. Biophys. Acta* **2013**, *1830*, 3289–3303. [CrossRef] [PubMed]
26. Jerome-Morais, A.; Bera, S.; Rachidi, W.; Gann, P.H.; Diamond, A.M. The effects of selenium and the GPx-1 selenoprotein on the phosphorylation of H2AX. *Biochim. Biophys. Acta* **2013**, *1830*, 3399–3406. [CrossRef] [PubMed]
27. Chen, X.; Fu, G.; Li, L.; Zhao, Q.; Ke, Z.; Zhang, R. Selenoprotein GPX1 is a prognostic and chemotherapy-related biomarker for brain lower grade glioma. *J. Trace Elem. Med. Biol.* **2022**, *74*, 127082. [CrossRef]
28. Schmidlin, C.J.; Shakya, A.; Dodson, M.; Chapman, E.; Zhang, D.D. The intricacies of NRF2 regulation in cancer. *Semin. Cancer Biol.* **2021**, *76*, 110–119. [CrossRef]
29. Bartolini, D.; Tew, K.D.; Marinelli, R.; Galli, F.; Wang, G.Y. Nrf2-modulation by seleno-hormetic agents and its potential for radiation protection. *BioFactors* **2020**, *46*, 239–245. [CrossRef]
30. Bao, Y.P.; Jemth, P.; Mannervik, B.; Williamson, G. Reduction of thymine hydroperoxide by phospholipid hydroperoxide glutathione peroxidase and glutathione transferases. *Febs Lett.* **1997**, *410*, 210–212. [CrossRef]
31. Hu, Q.; Zhang, Y.; Lou, H.; Ou, Z.; Liu, J.; Duan, W.; Wang, H.; Ge, Y.; Min, J.; Wang, F.; et al. GPX4 and vitamin E cooperatively protect hematopoietic stem and progenitor cells from lipid peroxidation and ferroptosis. *Cell Death Dis.* **2021**, *12*, 706. [CrossRef] [PubMed]
32. Yant, L.J.; Ran, Q.T.; Rao, L.; Van Remmen, H.; Shibatani, T.; Belter, J.G.; Motta, L.; Richardson, A.; Prolla, T.A. The selenoprotein GPX4 is essential for mouse development and protects from radiation and oxidative damage insults. *Free Radic. Biol. Med.* **2003**, *34*, 496–502. [CrossRef]
33. Liang, H.; Ran, Q.; Jang, Y.C.; Holstein, D.; Lechleiter, J.; McDonald-Marsh, T.; Musatov, A.; Song, W.; Van Remmen, H.; Richardson, A. Glutathione peroxidase 4 differentially regulates the release of apoptogenic proteins from mitochondria. *Free Radic. Biol. Med.* **2009**, *47*, 312–320. [CrossRef]
34. Huang, X.; Yang, X.; Zhang, M.; Li, T.; Zhu, K.; Dong, Y.; Lei, X.; Yu, Z.; Lv, C.; Huang, J. SELENOI Functions as a Key Modulator of Ferroptosis Pathway in Colitis and Colorectal Cancer. *Adv. Sci.* **2024**, *11*, e2404073. [CrossRef] [PubMed]
35. Schomburg, L. Selenoprotein P—Selenium transport protein, enzyme and biomarker of selenium status. *Free Radic. Biol. Med.* **2022**, *191*, 150–163. [CrossRef] [PubMed]
36. Eckers, J.C.; Kalen, A.L.; Xiao, W.S.; Sarsour, E.H.; Goswami, P.C. Selenoprotein P Inhibits Radiation-Induced Late Reactive Oxygen Species Accumulation and Normal Cell Injury. *Int. J. Radiat. Oncol. Biol. Phys.* **2013**, *87*, 619–625. [CrossRef] [PubMed]
37. Fisher, C.J.; Goswami, P.C. Mitochondria-targeted antioxidant enzyme activity regulates radioresistance in human pancreatic cancer cells. *Cancer Biol. Thera.* **2008**, *7*, 1271–1279. [CrossRef] [PubMed]
38. Kalen, A.L.; Sarsour, E.H.; Venkataraman, S.; Goswami, P.C. Mn-superoxide dismutase overexpression enhances G_2 accumulation and radioresistance in human oral squamous carcinoma cells. *Antiox. Redox Signaling* **2006**, *8*, 1273–1281. [CrossRef]
39. Barrett, C.W.; Reddy, V.K.; Short, S.P.; Motley, A.K.; Lintel, M.K.; Bradley, A.M.; Freeman, T.; Vallance, J.; Ning, W.; Parang, B.; et al. Selenoprotein P influences colitis-induced tumorigenesis by mediating stemness and oxidative damage. *J. Clin. Investig.* **2015**, *125*, 2646–2660. [CrossRef]
40. Vunta, H.; Belda, B.J.; Arner, R.J.; Reddy, C.C.; Heuvel, J.P.V.; Prabhu, K.S. Selenium attenuates pro-inflammatory gene expression in macrophages. *Mol. Nutr. Food Res.* **2008**, *52*, 1316–1323. [CrossRef]
41. Carlson, B.A.; Yoo, M.H.; Shrimali, R.K.; Irons, R.; Gladyshev, V.N.; Hatfield, D.L.; Park, J.M. Session 2: Micronutrients and the immune system Role of selenium-containing proteins in T-cell and macrophage function. *Proc. Nutr. Soc.* **2010**, *69*, 300–310. [CrossRef]
42. Jing, J.; He, Y.; Liu, Y.; Tang, J.; Wang, L.; Jia, G.; Liu, G.; Chen, X.; Tian, G.; Cai, J.; et al. Selenoproteins synergistically protect porcine skeletal muscle from oxidative damage via relieving mitochondrial dysfunction and endoplasmic reticulum stress. *J. Anim. Sci. Biotechnol.* **2023**, *14*, 79. [CrossRef] [PubMed]
43. Ghelichkhani, F.; Gonzalez, F.A.; Kapitonova, M.A.; Schaefer-Ramadan, S.; Liu, J.; Cheng, R.J.; Rozovsky, S. Selenoprotein S: A versatile disordered protein. *Arch. Biochem. Biophys.* **2022**, *731*, 109427. [CrossRef] [PubMed]
44. Huang, X.; Li, T.; Yang, S.H.; Zhu, K.D.; Wang, L.S.; Dong, Y.L.; Huang, J.Q. Hepatocyte-specific Selenoi deficiency predisposes mice to hepatic steatosis and obesity. *FASEB J.* **2024**, *38*, e23717. [CrossRef] [PubMed]

45. Ma, C.; Martinez-Rodriguez, V.; Hoffmann, P.R. Roles for Selenoprotein I and Ethanolamine Phospholipid Synthesis in T Cell Activation. *Int. J. Mol. Sci.* **2021**, *22*, 11174. [CrossRef] [PubMed]
46. Fu, G.; Guy, C.S.; Chapman, N.M.; Palacios, G.; Wei, J.; Zhou, P.; Long, L.; Wang, Y.D.; Qian, C.; Dhungana, Y.; et al. Metabolic control of T(FH) cells and humoral immunity by phosphatidylethanolamine. *Nature* **2021**, *595*, 724–729. [CrossRef]
47. Gorrini, C.; Harris, I.S.; Mak, T.W. Modulation of oxidative stress as an anticancer strategy. *Nat. Rev. Drug Discov.* **2013**, *12*, 931–947. [CrossRef]
48. Stein, T.P. Space flight and oxidative stress. *Nutrition* **2002**, *18*, 867–871. [CrossRef]
49. Fattman, C.L.; Schaefer, L.M.; Oury, T.D. Extracellular superoxide dismutase in biology and medicine. *Free Radic. Biol. Med.* **2003**, *35*, 236–256. [CrossRef]
50. Kiełczykowska, M.; Kocot, J.; Paździor, M.; Musik, I. Selenium—A fascinating antioxidant of protective properties. *Adv. Clin. Exp. Med.* **2018**, *27*, 245–255. [CrossRef]
51. Weiss, J.F.; Srinivasan, V.; Kumar, K.S.; Landauer, M.R. Radioprotection by metals: Selenium. *Adv. Space Res.* **1992**, *12*, 223–231. [CrossRef] [PubMed]
52. Ushakova, T.; Melkonyan, H.; Nikonova, L.; Afanasyev, V.; Gaziev, A.I.; Mudrik, N.; Bradbury, R.; Gogvadze, V. Modification of gene expression by dietary antioxidants in radiation-induced apoptosis of mice splenocytes. *Free Radic. Biol. Med.* **1999**, *26*, 887–891. [CrossRef] [PubMed]
53. De Haan, J.B.; Crack, P.J.; Flentjar, N.; Iannello, R.C.; Hertzog, P.J.; Kola, I. An imbalance in antioxidant defense affects cellular function: The pathophysiological consequences of a reduction in antioxidant defense in the glutathione peroxidase-1 (Gpx1) knockout mouse. *Redox Rep.* **2003**, *8*, 69–79. [CrossRef] [PubMed]
54. Shimizu, I.; Yoshida, Y.; Suda, M.; Minamino, T. DNA damage response and metabolic disease. *Cell Metab.* **2014**, *20*, 967–977. [CrossRef]
55. Bera, S.; De Rosa, V.; Rachidi, W.; Diamond, A.M. Does a role for selenium in DNA damage repair explain apparent controversies in its use in chemoprevention? *Mutagenesis* **2013**, *28*, 127–134. [CrossRef]
56. Zeng, H.; Davis, C.D.; Finley, J.W. Effect of selenium-enriched broccoli diet on differential gene expression in min mouse liver(1,2). *J. Nutr. Biochem.* **2003**, *14*, 227–231. [CrossRef]
57. Fischer, J.L.; Lancia, J.K.; Mathur, A.; Smith, M.L. Selenium protection from DNA damage involves a Ref1/p53/Brca1 protein complex. *Anticancer Res.* **2006**, *26*, 899–904.
58. Yan, Y.Q.; Liu, M.; Xu, Z.J.; Xu, Z.J.; Huang, Y.X.; Li, X.M.; Chen, C.J.; Zuo, G.; Yang, J.C.; Lei, X.G.; et al. Optimum Doses and Forms of Selenium Maintaining Reproductive Health via Regulating Homeostasis of Gut Microbiota and Testicular Redox, Inflammation, Cell Proliferation, and Apoptosis in Roosters. *J. Nutr.* **2024**, *154*, 369–380. [CrossRef]
59. Yang, S.; Huang, J.; Liu, P.; Li, J.; Zhao, S. Apoptosis-inducing factor (AIF) nuclear translocation mediated caspase-independent mechanism involves in X-ray-induced MCF-7 cell death. *Int. J. Radiat. Biol.* **2017**, *93*, 270–278. [CrossRef]
60. Hariharan, S.; Dharmaraj, S. Selenium and selenoproteins: It's role in regulation of inflammation. *Inflammopharmacology* **2020**, *28*, 667–695. [CrossRef]
61. Jiao, Y.; Cao, F.; Liu, H. Radiation-induced Cell Death and Its Mechanisms. *Health Phys.* **2022**, *123*, 376–386. [CrossRef] [PubMed]
62. Huang, J.Q.; Jiang, Y.Y.; Ren, F.Z.; Lei, X.G. Novel role and mechanism of glutathione peroxidase-4 in nutritional pancreatic atrophy of chicks induced by dietary selenium deficiency. *Redox Biol.* **2022**, *57*, 102482. [CrossRef] [PubMed]
63. Kaur, M.; Drake, A.C.; Hu, G.; Rudnick, S.; Chen, Q.; Phennicie, R.; Attar, R.; Nemeth, J.; Gaudet, F.; Chen, J. Induction and Therapeutic Targeting of Human NPM1c(+) Myeloid Leukemia in the Presence of Autologous Immune System in Mice. *J. Immunol.* **2019**, *202*, 1885–1894. [CrossRef] [PubMed]
64. Liu, C.; Wang, Z.; Wang, W.; Zheng, L.; Li, M. Positive effects of selenium supplementation on selenoprotein S expression and cytokine status in a murine model of acute liver injury. *J. Trace Elem. Med. Biol.* **2022**, *71*, 126927. [CrossRef]
65. Lu, M.; Wang, Y.; Zhan, X. The MAPK Pathway-Based Drug Therapeutic Targets in Pituitary Adenomas. *Front. Endocrinol.* **2019**, *10*, 330. [CrossRef]
66. Wang, J.; Shao, W.; Niu, H.; Yang, T.; Wang, Y.; Cai, Y. Immunomodulatory Effects of Colistin on Macrophages in Rats by Activating the p38/MAPK Pathway. *Front. Pharmacol.* **2019**, *10*, 729. [CrossRef]
67. Wang, Y.; Li, X.; Yao, Y.; Zhao, X.; Shi, X.; Cai, Y. Selenium Deficiency Induces Apoptosis and Necroptosis Through ROS/MAPK Signal in Human Uterine Smooth Muscle Cells. *Biol. Trace Elem. Res.* **2022**, *200*, 3147–3158. [CrossRef]
68. Toulany, M.; Rodemann, H.P. Phosphatidylinositol 3-kinase/Akt signaling as a key mediator of tumor cell responsiveness to radiation. *Semin. Cancer Biol.* **2015**, *35*, 180–190. [CrossRef]
69. Wang, S.; Liu, Y.; Sun, Q.; Zeng, B.; Liu, C.; Gong, L.; Wu, H.; Chen, L.; Jin, M.; Guo, J.; et al. Triple Cross-linked Dynamic Responsive Hydrogel Loaded with Selenium Nanoparticles for Modulating the Inflammatory Microenvironment via PI3K/Akt/NF-κB and MAPK Signaling Pathways. *Adv. Sci.* **2023**, *10*, e2303167. [CrossRef]
70. Yahyapour, R.; Amini, P.; Rezapour, S.; Cheki, M.; Rezaeyan, A.; Farhood, B.; Shabeeb, D.; Musa, A.E.; Fallah, H.; Najafi, M. Radiation-induced inflammation and autoimmune diseases. *Mil. Med. Res.* **2018**, *5*, 9. [CrossRef]
71. Molinar-Inglis, O.; DiCarlo, A.L.; Lapinskas, P.J.; Rios, C.I.; Satyamitra, M.M.; Silverman, T.A.; Winters, T.A.; Cassatt, D.R. Radiation-induced multi-organ injury. *Int. J. Radiat. Biol.* **2024**, *100*, 486–504. [CrossRef] [PubMed]
72. Mahmood, J.; Jelveh, S.; Calveley, V.; Zaidi, A.; Doctrow, S.R.; Hill, R.P. Mitigation of lung injury after accidental exposure to radiation. *Radiat. Res.* **2011**, *176*, 770–780. [CrossRef] [PubMed]

73. Sieber, F.; Muir, S.A.; Cohen, E.P.; North, P.E.; Fish, B.L.; Irving, A.A.; Mader, M.; Moulder, J.E. High-Dose Selenium for the Mitigation of Radiation Injury: A Pilot Study in a Rat Model. *Radiat. Res.* **2009**, *171*, 368–373. [CrossRef] [PubMed]
74. Kunwar, A.; Jain, V.K.; Priyadarsini, K.I.; Haston, C.K. A selenocysteine derivative therapy affects radiation-induced pneumonitis in the mouse. *Am. J. Respir. Cell Mol. Biol.* **2013**, *49*, 654–661. [CrossRef] [PubMed]
75. Cruz, L.Y.; Wang, D.; Liu, J. Biosynthesis of selenium nanoparticles, characterization and X-ray induced radiotherapy for the treatment of lung cancer with interstitial lung disease. *J. Photochem. Photobiol. B.* **2019**, *191*, 123–127. [CrossRef]
76. Zhang, J.; Han, Y.F.; Song, M.; Wang, Q.; Cao, Z.; Yang, X.; Li, Y.F. Selenium Improves Bone Microenvironment-Related Hematopoiesis and Immunity in T-2 Toxin-Exposed Mice. *J. Agric. Food Chem.* **2023**, *71*, 2590–2599. [CrossRef]
77. Li, T.; Zhu, K.; Wang, L.; Dong, Y.; Huang, J. Stabilization by Chaperone GroEL in Biogenic Selenium Nanoparticles Produced from Bifidobacterium animalis H15 for the Treatment of DSS-Induced Colitis. *ACS Appl. Mater. Interfaces* **2024**, *16*, 13439–13452. [CrossRef]
78. Short, S.P.; Pilat, J.M.; Barrett, C.W.; Reddy, V.K.; Haberman, Y.; Hendren, J.R.; Marsh, B.J.; Keating, C.E.; Motley, A.K.; Hill, K.E.; et al. Colonic Epithelial-Derived Selenoprotein P Is the Source for Antioxidant-Mediated Protection in Colitis-Associated Cancer. *Gastroenterology* **2021**, *160*, 1694–1708.e1693. [CrossRef]
79. Karami, M.; Asri-Rezaei, S.; Dormanesh, B.; Nazarizadeh, A. Comparative study of radioprotective effects of selenium nanoparticles and sodium selenite in irradiation-induced nephropathy of mice model. *Int. J. Radiat. Biol.* **2018**, *94*, 17–27. [CrossRef]
80. El-Ghazaly, M.A.; Fadel, N.; Rashed, E.; El-Batal, A.; Kenawy, S.A. Anti-inflammatory effect of selenium nanoparticles on the inflammation induced in irradiated rats. *Can. J. Physiol. Pharmacol.* **2017**, *95*, 101–110. [CrossRef]
81. Fahmy, H.A.; Abd El Azim, A.S.; Gharib, O.A. Protective Effects of ω-3 fatty acids and/or Nano- selenium on Cisplatin and Ionizing radiation induced liver toxicity in rats. *Indian J. Pharm. Educ. Res.* **2016**, *50*, 649–656. [CrossRef]
82. Azmoonfar, R.; Moslehi, M.; Shahbazi-Gahrouei, D. Radioprotective Effect of Selenium Nanoparticles: A Mini Review. *IET Nanobiotechnol.* **2024**, *2024*, 5538107. [CrossRef] [PubMed]
83. Musa, A.E.; Shabeeb, D. Radiation-Induced Heart Diseases: Protective Effects of Natural Products. *Medicina* **2019**, *55*, 126. [CrossRef]
84. Xiong, Y.; Liu, X.W.; Lee, C.P.; Chua, B.H.L.; Ho, Y.S. Attenuation of doxorubicin-induced contractile and mitochondrial dysfunction in mouse heart by cellular glutathione peroxidase. *Free Radic. Biol. Med.* **2006**, *41*, 46–55. [CrossRef]
85. Gao, J.P.; Xiong, Y.; Ho, Y.S.; Liu, X.W.; Chua, C.C.; Xu, X.S.; Wang, H.; Hamdy, R.; Chua, B.H.L. Glutathione peroxidase 1-deficient mice are more susceptible to doxorubicin-induced cardiotoxicity. *Biochim. Biophys. Acta, Mol. Cell Res.* **2008**, *1783*, 2020–2029. [CrossRef] [PubMed]
86. Lippman, S.M.; Klein, E.A.; Goodman, P.J.; Lucia, M.S.; Thompson, I.M.; Ford, L.G.; Parnes, H.L.; Minasian, L.M.; Gaziano, J.M.; Hartline, J.A.; et al. Effect of selenium and vitamin E on risk of prostate cancer and other cancers: The Selenium and Vitamin E Cancer Prevention Trial (SELECT). *JAMA* **2009**, *301*, 39–51. [CrossRef] [PubMed]
87. Shamberger, R.J.; Frost, D.V. Possible protective effect of selenium against human cancer. *Can. Med. Assoc. J.* **1969**, *100*, 682.
88. Waters, D.J.; Shen, S.; Glickman, L.T.; Cooley, D.M.; Bostwick, D.G.; Qian, J.; Combs, G.F., Jr.; Morris, J.S. Prostate cancer risk and DNA damage: Translational significance of selenium supplementation in a canine model. *Carcinogenesis* **2005**, *26*, 1256–1262. [CrossRef]
89. Liu, H.; Xu, H.; Huang, K. Selenium in the prevention of atherosclerosis and its underlying mechanisms. *Metallomics* **2017**, *9*, 21–37. [CrossRef]
90. Wu, M.; Kang, M.M.; Schoene, N.W.; Cheng, W.H. Selenium compounds activate early barriers of tumorigenesis. *J. Biol. Chem.* **2010**, *285*, 12055–12062. [CrossRef]
91. Wang, Y.; Jiang, L.; Li, Y.; Luo, X.; He, J. Effect of Different Selenium Supplementation Levels on Oxidative Stress, Cytokines, and Immunotoxicity in Chicken Thymus. *Biol. Trace Elem. Res.* **2016**, *172*, 488–495. [CrossRef] [PubMed]
92. Sánchez-Gutiérrez, M.; García-Montalvo, E.A.; Izquierdo-Vega, J.A.; Del Razo, L.M. Effect of dietary selenium deficiency on the in vitro fertilizing ability of mice spermatozoa. *Cell Biol. Toxicol.* **2008**, *24*, 321–329. [CrossRef] [PubMed]
93. Zhou, J.C.; Zheng, S.; Mo, J.; Liang, X.; Xu, Y.; Zhang, H.; Gong, C.; Liu, X.L.; Lei, X.G. Dietary Selenium Deficiency or Excess Reduces Sperm Quality and Testicular mRNA Abundance of Nuclear Glutathione Peroxidase 4 in Rats. *J. Nutr.* **2017**, *147*, 1947–1953. [CrossRef] [PubMed]
94. Zhang, Y.; Liu, J.; Li, X.; Zhou, G.; Sang, Y.; Zhang, M.; Gao, L.; Xue, J.; Zhao, M.; Yu, H.; et al. Dietary selenium excess affected spermatogenesis via DNA damage and telomere-related cell senescence and apoptosis in mice. *Food Chem. Toxicol.* **2023**, *171*, 113556. [CrossRef]

MDPI AG
Grosspeteranlage 5
4052 Basel
Switzerland
Tel.: +41 61 683 77 34

Nutrients Editorial Office
E-mail: nutrients@mdpi.com
www.mdpi.com/journal/nutrients

www.ingramcontent.com/pod-product-compliance
Lightning Source LLC
Chambersburg PA
CBHW062058220926
51850CB00010B/2811
* 9 7 8 3 7 2 5 8 7 6 6 1 7 *